FORENSIC TOXICOLOGY
FOR THE
LAW ENFORCEMENT OFFICER

Forensic Toxicology
For the
Law Enforcement Officer

By

CHARLES G. WILBER, Ph.D.

Fellow, American Academy of Forensic Sciences
Former Deputy Coroner
Larimer County, Colorado
Director, Forensic Science Laboratory
Colorado State University
Fort Collins, Colorado

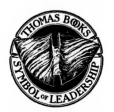

CHARLES C THOMAS · PUBLISHER
Springfield · Illinois · U.S.A.

Published and Distributed Throughout the World by
CHARLES C THOMAS • PUBLISHER
BANNERSTONE HOUSE
301-327 East Lawrence Avenue, Springfield, Illinois, U.S.A.

© *1980 by* CHARLES C THOMAS • PUBLISHER
ISBN 0-398-03922-4
Library of Congress Catalog Card Number: 79-12327

With THOMAS BOOKS *careful attention is given to all details of*
manufacturing and design. It is the Publisher's desire to present
books that are satisfactory as to their physical qualities and artistic
possibilities and appropriate for their particular use. THOMAS
BOOKS *will be true to those laws of quality that assure a good*
name and good will.

Printed in the United States of America
N-11

Library of Congress Cataloging in Publication Data

Wilber, Charles Grady, 1916-
    Forensic toxicology for the law enforcement officer.

    Bibliography: p.
    Includes index.
    1. Forensic toxicology.   2. Criminal investigation.
I. Title.
RA1228.W54   614'.19   79-12327
ISBN 0-398-03922-4

PREFACE

L AW ENFORCEMENT officers in the United States and in other nations from time to time are faced with crimes that involve the use of chemicals having adverse effects on the human body, that is, poisons. In the United States, the use of poisons as instruments of homicide is not frequent. Accidental poisonings and suicidal poisonings are more common. In other countries of the world, poisons are more commonly used for homicidal purposes.

Environmental poisonings associated with employment can strike at police officers as well as other automobile drivers in the form of carbon monoxide leaking into an automobile passenger compartment. When emergencies arise as a result of industrial poisonings, suicides, carrier accidents on the highways or on the rails, and related crises resulting in the release of poisonous (toxic) materials into man's surroundings, the police are the first personnel to be called on the scene. It therefore behooves them to have a reasonably detailed and extensive knowledge of various poisonous substances and what to do about protecting themselves and others from those substances.

This book is intended to be an introduction to the science of poisons. It is not intended that it be an encyclopedic volume for the research toxicologist, although he may find it a ready reference for many poisoning questions. The book is designed for the law enforcement officer, security man, and others in the criminal justice system, as a reference that can be easily read to provide the basic concepts of poisons, poisonings, and what to do about them.

Professors in police science or forensic science may find the book a convenient text to use. Attorneys, coroners, medical examiners, and judges will find the book a ready reference that may be adequate for their requirements in many cases.

In the finishing of any book manuscript, there are those heroic persons who read the author's scribble or listen to his interminable tapes and transform them into an acceptable typescript. I am deeply in debt to such a team of professionals in the office of the Department of Zoology-Entomology, Colorado State University. My warm thanks for a job well done go to Mary Wright, Gayle Roslund, Marilyn Pfaff, and Reta Herbertson.

I am also grateful for the atmosphere created at Colorado State University, which stimulates scholarly endeavor. Dr. Charles Ralph, Chairman of the Department of Zoology-Entomology, deserves great credit for insuring such a climate within that department.

Many colleagues and commercial firms have provided illustrative material with permission to publish it. Acknowledgments have been made at appropriate points in the text. Many sympathetic persons have responded generously to my requests for help. I wish I could thank them individually for their favors.

I also acknowledge with warm thanks and personal pleasure the efforts of my wife, Clare Marie Wilber, in proofreading the galleys and the page proofs.

CHARLES G. WILBER

INTRODUCTION

E ACH YEAR from all parts of the world, more than 1 million persons are acutely poisoned in some manner or other. There are at least 50,000 poisonous materials that can be purchased "over the counter" by the ordinary citizen for various valid uses. Some of these materials can (and do) cause accidental poisonings in man. A few are used by unfortunates bent on suicide. Fewer still serve as murder weapons for criminals.

The latter use of toxic materials is of continuing interest to all law enforcement personnel. The insidiousness and maliciousness of the use of poisons for deliberate homicide make these agents a challenge to investigators and forensic toxicologists.

The subject of forensic toxicology is complex; its practitioners require rigorous technical training, broad education, plus demanding practical experience in order to function effectively in our criminal justice system. Law enforcement officers need an understanding of toxicology, what it is, and how toxicologists can contribute to the solution of criminal cases.

Moreover, the realm of forensic toxicology of necessity is no longer limited to criminal proceedings. Environmental toxicology, occupational toxicology, and pesticide toxicology are becoming more prominent in the legal process through hearings, panels, civil suits, liability, environmental impact statements, and numerous other kinds of litigation so dear to the heart of America. The forensic aspects of toxicology are needed in these new activities; the level of expert testimony in these subjects is dismal at the moment.

An Example

The need for a generalized knowledge of toxicology by law enforcement officers is illustrated by a recent death that occurred in a western state, where poisonings are even more rare than in many other parts of the country.

> A young man, nineteen years of age, was found dead in an isolated dwelling. There was no sign of violence, nor were there any obvious indications that the death was from other than natural causes. Fortunately, one of the officers investigating the case detected the smell of "burnt almonds" or peach stones in the vicinity of the body. (He admitted to being an avid reader of high-quality detective stories and remembered several in which the bitter almond smell was a clue.) This observation, recorded in his report, suggested death by other than natural causes. A thorough autopsy was therefore ordered by the local coroner; death by ingestion of cyanide (used in coyote bait) was confirmed. Careful police investigation of all the attending circumstances proved that the death was suicidal.

A matter of considerable concern is the high probability that had the deceased been an elderly person rather than a youth, nine times out of ten the death would have been declared "natural" and no postmortem examination would have been ordered.

Some of the signs observed in victims of poisons are associated with bacterial diseases. Crime scene investigators need sufficient knowledge of poisons to be able to raise a suspicion when faced with clues that may signal the presence of some toxic substance as the cause of death.

Poison Deaths

Poison deaths most commonly encountered by the investigating officer are associated with drugs of abuse. In certain seasons of the year in some parts of the United States, deaths from carbon monoxide poisoning may be more prevalent. Drug deaths and carbon monoxide deaths are usually either accidental or suicidal. Despite interesting stories of "hot shots" (excessively pure samples of a drug like heroin given to an addict without his knowledge) being used to eliminate an addict for some reason, the documented cases of such happenings are meager.

Murder by poisoning in the United States is extremely rare. Homicide by poison is by its very nature difficult to prove. The problem of associating a specific suspect with the actual administration of a fatal dose of a proven poison is not readily solved. Investigative techniques in poison cases require special attention, particularly in the collection and storage of evidence and in the recording of detailed collateral information to be given to the toxicologist doing the poison analyses.*

The Autopsy

Death by poison, no matter what the manner may be, underlines the need for a thorough autopsy in every case of death where violence is not obvious but natural causes seem vague. Moreover, where death is of undetermined cause, it is unacceptable that an autopsy not be done. When in doubt, toxicological tests should be run to at least reveal a general class of poison that might be involved.

Household Medicines

Medicines are important in the control of disease in children and in adults. However, when inadequately controlled, medicines themselves cause harm, especially in children. There are data to show that several million children five years old or less face accidental poisoning each year. Common aspirin is involved in well over one-third of the cases. The so-called child-proof medicine containers may be useful in homes where there are young children, but persons with arthritis involving the hand and fingers may find such containers impossible to open in an emergency. In the absence of children, adults who need regular medicines or who may require emergency medicines should have the trick stoppers removed and thrown away. The container can then be stoppered with a cork of suitable size.

First Aid

There are a number of basic principles law enforcement officers should remember with respect to first aid treatment of

---

*A case in 1978 of alleged poisoning with curare should be kept in mind because the judge refused to let the jury hear toxicological evidence unless poison was demonstrated by two separate, distinct, and independent corroborating tests that were accepted by scientists as valid (Bird, 1978).

poisonings. If the victim is conscious and has not swallowed an irritating poison or one that is corrosive, every effort should be made to empty the subject's stomach by causing vomiting; washing out the stomach (gastric lavage) is strictly a medical procedure and should not be attempted by the police officer.

The simplest method to cause vomiting is to push a finger down the victim's throat, pressing the tip of the finger gently toward the front of the body. In many instances that maneuver is sufficient to bring about the vomiting reflex.

If vomiting does not result from that simple procedure, a small amount of *syrup of ipecac* may be given. A dose of ½ teaspoonful should cause a child to vomit in about 15 minutes. Several glasses of water help the vomiting to develop. Most children older than a year or two can be given 1 teaspoonful for smaller children; up to 3 teaspoonfuls of ipecac are useful for adults. If vomiting does not occur in 20 minutes, the dose may be repeated but ONLY ONCE MORE. More ipecac than recommended can itself be toxic.

After the stomach is emptied as completely as possible by vomiting, the remaining poison in the stomach can be absorbed by *activated charcoal*. A dose of 2 rounded tablespoons of the charcoal powder is mixed in the tumbler with enough water to make a solution that is easy to drink. The mixture should be given to the victim regularly until medical attention is on the scene.

Vomiting is *not* to be induced if the victim has swallowed a corrosive poison (lye, acids) or volatiles such as gasoline, kerosene, cleaning fluid, turpentine, or petroleum products in general. Vomiting after the swallowing of these poisons is extremely dangerous for the victim. Soothing agents should be given: milk, egg white, aluminum hydroxide gel, gelatin solution, or flour and water slurry. IMMEDIATE MEDICAL ATTENTION IN A HOSPITAL IS ESSENTIAL.

Commercially available poison antidote kits containing activated charcoal, ipecac, and instructions are on the market. Figure I-1 illustrates one of these poison antidote kits.

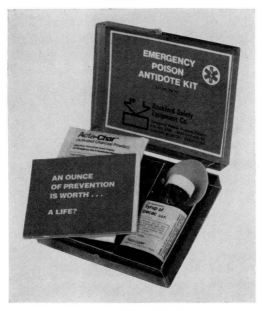

Figure I-1. This commercially available emergency poison antidote kit is simple and easy enough for use by nonmedical personnel. The kit contains a list of measures to help prevent accidental poisoning; instructions on what to do when poisoning occurs; one packet of Acta-Char™ (activated charcoal powder) 0.35 oz. net wt. (10 gm); complete chart showing types of poisons and correct counterdoses; a 1 oz. bottle of syrup of ipecac; and a plastic tablespoon. Size is 4 by 5¼ by 1½ inches. Courtesy of Rockford Safety Equipment Company, Rockford, Illinois.

The PK-10 Antidote Kit provides effective first aid so poisons cannot work unchecked. The kit is not intended as final treatment but as a lifesaving first aid measure. The two antidotes, syrup of ipecac and activated charcoal, are easily administered as early treatment in accidental poisoning. Syrup of ipecac is an integral part of the kit and causes vomiting. Acta-Char™ is included to neutralize or absorb the poison. If neither antidote is indicated for the poison taken, a chart instructs the officer or "good Samaritan" what to give the victim immediately after the poisoning occurs and what to do until medical help is available. With these ingredients, the PK-10 Antidote Kit can be the difference, in many cases, between quick recovery and serious complications or even between life and death.

The relative toxicities of a number of household chemicals are shown in Table I-I.

Table I-I
MINIMUM LETHAL DOSE OF SOME REPRESENTATIVE HOUSEHOLD
MEDICINES*

Medicine	Minimum Lethal Dose
Acetanilid	4 gm
Amidopyrine	5 gm
Antipyrine	5 gm
Aspirin	20 gm
Boric acid	10 gm
Butazolidin®	5 gm
Camphor	2 gm
Methyl salicylate	20 ml
Phenacetin	5 gm
Phenol	10 ml
Darvon®	1 gm
Digitalis	3 gm
Dilantin®	5 gm
Doriden®†	5 gm
Dramamine®	50 mg/kg
Emetine	1 gm
Ephedrine	600 mg
Epinephrine (adrenaline)	100 mg
Ethclorvynol‡	15 gm
Isopropyl alcohol	240 ml
Menthol	2 gm

*(Simpson, 1967)

†Gluthethimide, also known as Doriden®, is a mild hypnotic that is useful as a substitute for barbiturates. At the time of arousal from drug overdose coma, the reported glutethimide content of the victim's blood serum varied from 4 to 18 mg/liter; the amounts in cerebrospinal fluid varied from 2 to 6 mg/liter (Gold et al., 1974).

‡The concentration of Placidyl®, or ethchlorvynol, in a patient frankly poisoned with the drug was at admission to treatment 5.6 to 6.0 ml/dl of blood; 120 hours after admission the concentration of drug had dropped to zero (Wallace et al., 1974).

Poisons and the Law

The law enforcement officer is primarily concerned with poisonings he will encounter in his usual professional activities.

These poisonings will be the result of suicide, accident, and in a small part, homicide. The spectrum of poisons he can anticipate in his work will necessarily be relatively narrow. Most of the suicides will probably result from the intake of barbiturates, the inhalation of auto exhaust fumes, or possibly in a few instances, the ingestion of excessive amounts of aspirinlike compounds.

Accidental poisonings will primarily involve household chemicals, including a variety of insecticides. There will, of course, be some accidents as a result of individuals being poisoned by carbon monoxide in automobiles with faulty exhaust systems or in dwellings having inadequate ventilation for the heating systems.

Homicidal poisonings are not common at this time in the United States, but the possibility that homicidal poisoning deaths are being missed is a matter that deserves serious consideration. Certain sophisticated poisons are difficult to identify (MacDonald, 1978). This book gives information that investigating officers, who are not toxicologists, can put into practice or use to reveal and uncover hidden poisoning deaths that may, in fact, go unrecognized up to this time.

Improving Expert Testimony

There has been thoughtful adverse criticism of the expert witness system as it operates in United States courts. MacDonald (1978), for example, uses the Coppolino trial in Florida to illustrate one problem. Dr. Carl Coppolino was charged with murdering his wife by injecting succinylcholine into her. Succinylcholine is a drug used by anesthesiologists for special purposes; it is a short-acting paralyzer of skeletal muscles.

There was a so-called battle of the experts who testified about the identification of succinylcholine in the wife's body and the interpretation of the results. The entire testimony was so technical and specialized that the jury was bewildered.

MacDonald suggests that, in cases such as these, expert testimony be condensed into a single informative statement for the court, couched in simple English, and based on a consensus between an expert appointed by the prosecution, one appointed by the defense, and a neutral referee agreed upon by both experts.

In the presence of the judge, opposing attorneys, and the two experts, the referee would present the consensus, which would be binding on court and adversaries. The plan could be used to advantage in civil cases. The proposal is worth serious consideration.

Administrative Law

There is another area of toxicology and the law that is a virtual quagmire of regulations, laws, and administrative decisions. This area includes the matter of drug abuse control and the control of pesticides and other types of materials that may be hazardous to individuals or groups under various conditions. Here are a few of the laws that, at the national level, involve toxicology and can truly be considered forensic toxicology: the Occupational Safety and Health Act of 1970, the Comprehensive Drug Abuse Prevention and Control Act of 1970, the Federal Food, Drug and Cosmetic Act as amended in January 1971, a series of acts controlling what materials are called hazardous substances, Child Protection and Toy Safety Act of 1969, Poison Prevention Packaging Act of 1970, and Public Health Cigarette Smoking Act of 1969. Then there is a whole series of laws such as Noise Pollution, Lead-Based Paint Poisoning Acts, Clear Air Act, Flammable Fabric Act, and so on. In order to administer these various federal laws, a bevy of governmental agencies is involved.

Some eleven major federal offices are charged with carrying out these activities. Within each of these offices are as many as ten or twelve subactivities. Consequently, toxicology for the law enforcement officer is merely part of the overall toxicological concern as represented in our federal and local laws. Many of the federal laws also contain devices that force state and local communities to enact comparable laws. Most of these laws are not enforced through the regular police agencies but have specific federal enforcement activities and officers provided in numbers that are hard to record.

Iatrogenic Poisoning

The term *iatrogenic poisoning* is used to refer to adverse reactions to drugs that are prescribed for a patient by a qualified physician. The term comes from two Greek words: *iatros,* meaning physician, and *gene,* meaning to produce. Iatrogenic poisoning may be an unavoidable hazard associated with the use of some treatment needed by the patient. In some cases, a patient has an idiosyncracy or personal peculiarity in his biological makeup that makes him uniquely and unpredictably sensitive to a therapeutic drug. For example, some individuals are extremely sensitive to aspirin and show severe toxic signs after even a single aspirin tablet. In most instances, iatrogenic poisoning must be accepted as a normal and proper risk associated with the use of any medical procedure aimed at curing a sick person.

In a small percentage of iatrogenic poisonings, there is the element of carelessness, ignorance, or incompetence. In these cases, ethical, civil, and even criminal considerations must be faced. It is these cases that may result quite properly in police investigation.

Reading through the various medical journals published in the United States discloses that a proportion of hospitalized patients in this country have bad drug reactions of such severity that their length of time in the hospital is doubled. Specifically, the patients have been poisoned by a given drug at a designated dosage schedule, or more commonly, by a dosage program involving several drugs administered simultaneously.

Overall, between 15 and 40 percent of all hospitalized patients have grave adverse drug reactions; that is, they show toxic signs and symptoms as a result of their treatment with drugs. Probably close to one-third of patients put into hospitals for medical problems develop at least one dangerous adverse drug reaction.

Claims of iatrogenic poisoning through the excessive use of tranquilizers in mental institutions in New York State have been aired. According to one medical examiner in that state, a large percentage of the deaths in at least two state mental health facilities are tranquilizer related. Reportedly, a number of these deaths involved patients who were so heavily drugged with tranquilizers that when they vomited from some cause, they drowned in their own vomit (Sullivan, 1978) .*

All the facts are not yet available in this situation. Nevertheless, these claims should alert law enforcement personnel to the possibility of such poisonings within their own jurisdictions. If public state-operated mental care facilities can be the locations of excessive drug giving by the staff, the question of private, loosely supervised mental institutions and rest homes presents itself. One of the causes of death to inmates of these facilities may be excessive medication, leading to frank drug toxicity or poisoning. Death investigators might keep in mind this possibility; if the suspicion arises, appropriate toxicological tests should be ordered.

National Referral Center

The Library of Congress is interested in registering all organizations, institutions, groups, or individuals with special knowledge or informational competence in any aspect of toxicology. This project is being undertaken by the National Referral Center for Science and Technology of the Library with support from the Toxicology Information Program of the National Library of Medicine. The purpose is to encourage the registration of all information resources on toxicology with the National Referral Center for Science and Technology. The data gathered will become a part of the Center's comprehensive register of information resources. The Center uses its current collection of over 8700 information resources to provide an ongoing referral service, directing those who need information on a particular subject to those organizations or individuals with specialized knowledge on that subject. The Center also issues directories covering both broad and specific subject fields and analyzes the nation's scientific information network.

Poison Control Centers

Virtually every community in the United States is located within an area served by a poison control center. Law enforce-

*"Among the prime contributors to the problem [of polydrug abuse] are doctors who are dispensing pills and prescriptions all too frequently" (Stockton, 1978).

ment agencies should have up-to-date addresses and phone numbers for these important support functions. If radio contact is available, the way to contact the center by radio should be in writing near all police radios. The following are some of the leading poison control centers listed regionally (Taylor, 1977).

New England

Poison Center
Children's Hospital Medical Center
300 Longwood Avenue
Boston, Massachusetts 02115
Telephone: (617) 232-2120

Vermont Poison Center
Medical Center Hospital of Vermont
Burlington, Vermont 05401
Telephone: (802) 656-2439

Middle Atlantic

Western New York Poison Center
Children's Hospital
219 Bryant Street
Buffalo, New York 14222
Telephone: (716) 878-7000

Poison Control Center
442 First Avenue
New York, New York 10016
Telephone: (212) 340-4494

Pittsburgh Poison Center
Children's Hospital of Pittsburgh
125 De Soto Street
Pittsburgh, Pennsylvania 15215
Telephone: (412) 681-6669

South

Poison Information Center
Children's Hospital
1601 Sixth Avenue South
Birmingham, Alabama 35233
Telephone: (205) 933-4050

Maryland Poison Information Center
University of Maryland at Baltimore
School of Pharmacy
636 West Lombard Street
Baltimore, Maryland 21201
Telephone: (301) 528-7701

Duke University Poison Control Center
Duke University Hospital
Durham, North Carolina 27710
Telephone: (919) 684-8111

Huntington Poison Center
St. Mary's Hospital
2900 First Avenue
Huntington, West Virginia 25701
Telephone: (304) 696-2224

Central

St. Louis Poison Center
Cardinal Glennon Memorial
  Hospital for Children
1465 South Grand Boulevard
St. Louis, Missouri 63104
Telephone: (314) 772-5200

Poison Information Center
Children's Memorial Hospital
44th Street and Dewey Avenue
Omaha, Nebraska 68104
Telephone: (402) 553-5400

Midwest

Poison Control Center
Children's Hospital of Michigan
3901 Beaubien Boulevard
Detroit, Michigan 48201
Telephone: (313)494-5711

Poison Information Center
Academy of Medicine of Cleveland
10525 Carnegie Avenue
Cleveland, Ohio 44106
Telephone: (216) 231-4455

Milwaukee Poison Center
Milwaukee Children's Hospital
1700 West Wisconsin Avenue
Milwaukee, Wisconsin 53233
Telephone: (414) 344-7100

Southwest

New Mexico Poison and Drug Infor-
  mation Center
Bernalillo County Medical Center
2211 Lomas Boulevard, N.E.
Albuquerque, New Mexico 87106
Telephone: (505) 843-2551

Poison Center
University of Texas Medical Branch
  Hospitals
8th Street and Mechanic Street
Galveston, Texas 77550
Telephone: (713) 765-1420

Rocky Mountain

Rocky Mountain Poison Center
Denver General Hospital
West 8th Avenue and Cherokee Street
Denver, Colorado 80204
Telephone: (303) 893-7771

Intermountain Regional Poison Con-
  trol Center
University of Utah Medical Center
50 North Medical Drive
Salt Lake City, Utah 84132
Telephone: (801) 581-2151

Pacific

Fairbanks Poison Center
Fairbanks Memorial Hospital
1650 Cowles Street
Fairbanks, Alaska 99701
Telephone: (907) 452-8181

Thomas J. Fleming Memorial Poison
  Information Center
Children's Hospital of Los Angeles
4650 Sunset Boulevard
Los Angeles, California 90027
Telephone: (206) 634-5252

Poison Information Center
Children's Orthopedic Hospital and
 Medical Center
4800 Sandpoint Way, N.E.
Seattle, Washington 98105
Telephone: (207) 634-5252

Chemical Emergencies

According to *The Police Chief* (official journal of the International Association of Chiefs of Police), round-the-clock help in chemical emergencies is available as quickly as you can make a telephone call.

Assistance in Chemical Emergencies

A national service supported by chemical manufacturers provides advice and assistance when a chemical spill, fire, or other incident involving chemicals occurs. CHEMTREC has a telephone central on duty twenty-four hours a day, seven days a week to handle toll-free calls (800/424-9300). Collect calls (415/233-3737) reach Chevron Chemical Company. In addition to telephone assistance, the National Agricultural Chemical Association has a ten-region network of safety teams to provide advice and, if necessary, to assist in handling the emergency.

Brochures giving general guidelines for handling personnel exposure, spills, and fires involving pesticides may be obtained upon request to Employee Relations/Safety, Chevron Chemical Company, P.O. Box 3744, San Francisco, California, 94119.

CONTENTS

FORENSIC TOXICOLOGY
FOR THE
LAW ENFORCEMENT OFFICER

Chapter 1

WHAT IS TOXICOLOGY?

The Art of the Poisoner

Poisoning has been used by man for murder and suicide as long as recorded history. Early in the sojourn of mankind on planet Earth, individual human beings learned that certain substances in the environment would cause severe illness and even death if taken into the body. The materials were recognized as originating from plants, animals, or the nonliving surroundings.

The Egyptians and the Greeks knew that certain plants had the capacity to inflict death on a victim. The Greek philosopher Socrates was executed by the state through the use of hemlock, a plant poison.

Around the year 200 B.C., a Greek handbook on poisons was written; it discussed in an informed way the poisonous qualities of opium, henbane, some fungi, aconite, and other substances. The author divided poisons into those that act quickly as opposed to those that act slowly.

In ancient India, the poisons arsenic, aconite, and opium were known. They were used by women to get rid of oppressive husbands. Thus it was that the practice of suttee, the burning of a widow on the husband's funeral pyre, was devised to curtail the elimination of unwanted husbands.

In Asia, there were said to be secret methods of slow poisoning. Could it be that the poisoning practitioner exposed his victim to the organism that causes smallpox? Or perhaps the poisoner gave his victim articles of clothing infected with typhus? We have no specific details.

"Ingenuity equal to that of any modern murderer was shown

3

by Parysatis, the wife of Darius the Persian, who killed Statira, the wife of Artaveres, by carving a bird with a knife smeared with poison on one side, so that one helping only was lethal" (Furneaux, 1957).

Practical women changed the art of poisoning into a profession. Locusta of Rome, a famous applied toxicologist, gave Agrippina poison with which to murder Emperor Claudius. From Locusta also came the poison that Nero used to eliminate Britannicus. In both instances, cyanide was probably used.

During the Middle Ages, arsenic, aconite, opium, strychnine, cyanide, and belladonna were of sustained popularity. These agents were used by professional poisoners into the sixteenth century in Italy and into the seventeenth century in France.

An early "Murder Incorporated" activity existed in the 1300s. In 1384, Charles the Bad, King of Navarre, let a contract for the King of France and his brothers to be "wasted," to use a current vulgarism. The contract specified that arsenic was to be used covertly.

Throughout Europe there was great fear of the poisoner who worked behind the scenes. In the fifteenth century, several Popes directed that dissections be done on the bodies of notables who died of unknown causes. This regulation was made in an attempt to reveal whether poison was used to bring about these deaths.

In the latter part of the eighteenth century, chemical science became sophisticated enough to provide useful chemical tests for poisons in human bodies. At that time, only inorganic or mineral poisons such as arsenic could be identified.

The first textbook on poison was written in 1814 by Matthew Joseph Orfila, who is considered to be the father of modern toxicology. In 1836 Marsh reported his test for arsenic. At the same time, new poisons, virtually undetectable by chemical testing, were being discovered or rediscovered and added to the murderer's arsenal of toxic agents. For example, the following poisons were introduced in the years indicated:

Morphine, 1803
Strychnine, 1818
Brucine, 1819

Codeine, 1832
Aconite, 1833

A Viewpoint

The poisoner is a murderer who has gone through a long and deliberate process of cold premeditation. A *homicidal* poisoning is a murder that has been precisely calculated. It is a crime as deliberate, as cold-blooded, as malicious, and as premeditated as is a covert bombing.

The Achilles' Heel of Murder

All murderers do evil deeds for some purpose; they kill for a specific reason. After they have murdered, they must gather their reward.

Most murderers kill someone close, a relative or an associate. Rarely is an unknown person killed. It is the trusted hand that wields the death blow. When the cause and manner of death are investigated, suspicions arise. A story given to the investigators fails to match the facts. Some persons, by training or shrewdness, may be able to create a more plausible story than others.

However, every murderer needs to reap the reward of his crime. The act of murder itself creates a new situation, an unfamiliar and unexpected role. When the murderer is then challenged, he stumbles, he attempts to ward off suspicion, and in the process he entangles himself.

How Insidious It Is

One of the characteristics of poisoning, whether on purpose or accidental, is its insidious nature, as illustrated by the following anecdote.

A representative of a foreign government was causing severe inroads into security and covert operations in a part of Europe. It was arranged for him to meet with a supposed government official in order to discuss further subversion. The "official" was an officer of the threatened country under a low-profile cover.

The meeting was held at a modest restaurant. The food was good and the coffee was excellent and plentiful. The next day there was another meeting; a modest meal, a small amount of wine, and a sheaf of documents passed over to the foreign representative from the "official." The two parted and the official disappeared. Back home, everyone knew he had taken a brief business trip to the nation's capital and had returned on schedule.

Two days after the final meeting of the pair, the foreign representative had flown to Vienna, where he suddenly became violently ill with nausea, vomiting, and diarrhea. He showed severe rhinitis and bronchitis. His eyes were bloodshot, and he had a temperature of about 100°F. His urine showed signs of kidney injury. Questioning him was useless because he was mentally confused.

He complained of severe pains in the back, arms, and legs. The feet could not tolerate even the touch of a sheet. He was in turn anxious, uneasy, and then delirious. His sleep pattern was erratic; the bronchitis became worse. In a week he was dead. At autopsy, the doctor noticed that the hair of the head, pubis, and axilla pulled out very easily. The diagnosis was severe polyneuritis complicated by fulminating pneumonia. Because the pathologist seemed so sure of his diagnosis, no chemical tests were performed on the tissues or body fluids of the deceased.

One part of the story was never known to the attending physician. During both meals with the victim, the official had excused himself "to visit the latrine." Instead he had spoken to the headwaiter about his friend's "diabetes," giving the headwaiter several tablets to put into the coffee and wine of his friend to counteract the excess sugar. He explained to the waiter that his friend was embarrassed about his condition and hated to make a public display of his disability. For a $10 bill each time, the cooperation of the headwaiter was insured.

The tablets were fast-dissolving forms of thallium acetate, a delayed-action poison. While the victim sickened, his "contact" was back home; by the time he died, the "contact" had almost forgotten the incident—no lasting thread tied the two together.

There are other poisons that can be used in a variety of ways for evildoing. Fortunately, the state of the art in analytical chemistry has advanced to a degree that virtually any poison can be identified quantitatively if adequate tests are run. It is true that there are still interfering substances that prevent some chemical analysis of bodily tissues. One of the most frustrating types of interference is the rapid embalming of a body that may have been subjected to a poison before death. The embalming procedure, including the chemicals used, interferes with many important chemical tests so as to render them useless. It is for this reason, among others, that forensic scientists are so strongly opposed to the rapid embalming of bodies of victims who may have died as a result of violence, under mysterious circumstances, or as a result of unknown causes. There is no reason for rapid embalming of bodies. Autopsies should be carried out on unembalmed bodies so that the tissues are not disturbed by the embalming process.

Toxicology as a Science

Toxicology is an offshoot of pharmacology or the study of drugs (Fig. 1-1). Toxicology is the science of poisons, their properties, isolation, purification, and quantitative estimation from biological material. This science includes the determination of lethal doses of chemicals, their action on living tissue, and the proper treatment to counteract the action of these harmful chemicals known as poisons.

Technically, a poison is practically any chemical substance given in a large enough dose. A useful definition is the following one: A poison is a substance that uniformly causes a disturbance of bodily function, injury, disease, or death when introduced into a living organism. The action of the poison is not mechanical but is primarily chemical in nature.

Another definition used to describe a poison is a substance that acts directly on the mucous membranes of the body, on other tissues of the body, or on the skin. The action may occur after absorption of the substance into the circulatory system to injure or destroy life in the body. The effect of such poison depends on how the poison is administered.

Forensic Toxicology

Forensic toxicology is the science of poisons and poisonings as related to the law. It is toxicology in the courtroom.

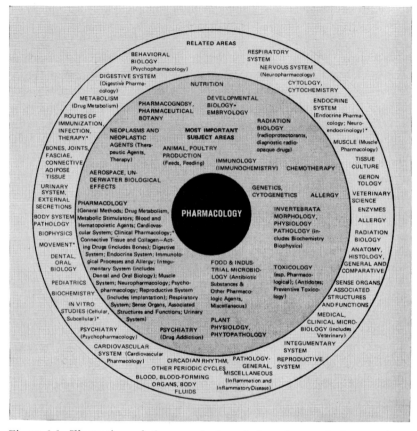

Figure 1-1. Illustration of the complexity of the science of pharmacology. Reproduced with permission of BioSciences Information Service, Philadelphia, Pennsylvania.

Toxicology is often included as a specialty within the field of pharmacology (the science of drugs and their actions in living organisms). Indeed, in many universities, the only toxicology taught is offered by the university department of pharmacology.

Toxicology itself is divided into a number of specialized areas: drugs and drug formulations, substances that cause dependence, foods and food additives, pesticides, industrial toxicology, environmental toxicology, forensic toxicology, military toxicology, and radiation toxicology (Fig. 1-2).

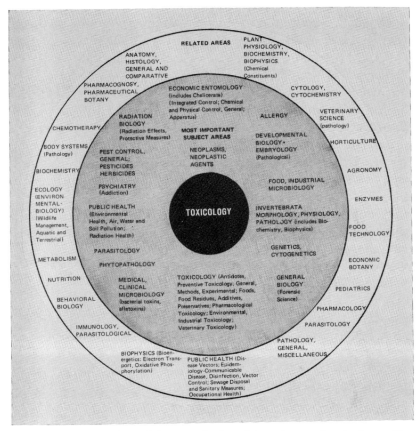

Figure 1-2. Illustration of the complexity of the science of toxicology. Reproduced with permission of BioSciences Information Service, Philadelphia, Pennsylvania.

For example, scientists who work with chemical warfare agents are military toxicologists. Those who work with the new neutron bomb are radiation toxicologists because the particles blasted about by the bomb are intensely radioactive; but they are also military toxicologists because of the chemical warfare effects of a shower of intense neutron radiation on the target, man.

One of the chief responsibilities of a toxicologist, an expert in the science of poisons, no matter whether he is with a law enforcement agency, a university, or some industrial laboratory, is what one might call prediction. The toxicologist must have a wealth of information on the mechanisms of action of various poisonous compounds so that he can predict or foresee the damage and effect that these poisonous agents will have on human individuals and human populations.*

Ariens, Simonis, and Offermeier (1976) have offered the following definition or description of forensic toxicology: "This area has to do with detection of poisons, often in postmortem material . . . where there is suspicion of murder or attempted murder by poisoning. Determination of blood alcohol concentration in expired air or blood and identification of suspicious substances in connection with trade in narcotics, as well as investigations on doping in sports, fall under this heading. These investigations are usually conducted in specially equipped forensic laboratories."

When simply defined as the science of poisons, toxicology is not represented in its true complexity (Fig. 1-2). Toxicology calls upon all the basic sciences in order to be effective. Thus, the expert toxicologist needs a broad background in the physical, chemical, and biological sciences if he is to be any more than a technician.

The Public Health Service (Christensen, 1973) defines, for inclusion in the *Toxic Substances List,* a toxic substance as follows:

> A toxic substance is one that demonstrates the potential to induce cancer, tumors, or neoplastic effects in man or experimental animals; to induce a permanent transmissible change in the characteristics of an offspring from those of its human or experimental animal parents; to cause the production of physical defects in the developing human or experimental animal embryo; to produce death in animals exposed via the respiratory tract, skin, eye, mouth, or other routes in quantities which are reasonable for experimental or domestic animals; to produce irritation or sensitization of the skin, eyes or respiratory passages; to diminish mental alertness, reduce motivation or alter behavior of humans; to adversely affect the health of a normal or disabled person of any age or of either sex by producing reversible or irreversible bod-

---

*Physicians and professional toxicologists will find much of interest and value in the technical publications of Comstock (1968), Hine, Hall, and Turkel (1968), and the Drug Enforcement Administration (1979).

ily injury or by endangering life or causing death from exposure via the respiratory tract, skin, eye, mouth, or any other route in any quantity, concentration, or dose reported for any length of time.

Some Terminology

As with any highly technical subject, toxicology has developed a specialized vocabulary of its own. In order to understand the basic facts of poisons and poisonings, it is essential to be familiar with the basic, specialized terminology used by toxicologists. With respect to the nature of the exposure to a poison, there are a number of useful terms. These have been taken directly from Christensen (1973).

These terms indicate whether the dose caused death (LD) or other toxic effects (TD) and whether it was administered as a lethal concentration (LC) or toxic concentration (TC) in the inhaled air. Their definitions are as follows:

TDLo: Toxic Dose Low. The lowest dose of a substance as published or made available to publish, introduced by any route, other than inhalation, over any given period of time and reported to produce any toxic effect in man or to produce carcinogenic, teratogenic, mutagenic, or neoplastigenic effects in humans or animals.

LDo: Lethal Dose Low. The lowest dose of a substance, other than LD_{50}, introduced by any route, other than inhalation, over any given period of time and reported to have caused death in man or the lowest single dose introduced in one or more divided portions and reported to have caused death in animals.

LD_{50}: Lethal Dose Fifty. A calculated dose of a chemical substance which is expected to cause the death of 50% of an entire population of an experimental animal species, as determined from the exposure to the substance, by any route other than inhalation, of a significant number from that population. Other lethal dose percentages, such as LD_1, LD_{10}, LD_{100}, as well as others, may be published in the scientific literature for the specific purposes of the author.

LCLo: Lethal Concentration Low. The lowest concentration of a substance, other than an LC_{50}, in air which has been reported to have caused death in man or to have caused death in animals when they have been exposed for twenty-four hours or less.

LC_{50}: Lethal Concentration Fifty. A calculated concentration of a substance in air to which exposure for twenty-four hours or less would cause the death of 50% of an entire population of an experimental animal species as determined from the exposure to the substance of a significant number from that population.

Units for Expressing Dosages

In most scientific studies of poisons, the doses (amounts taken in by the subject) are expressed as the amount or quantity of the toxic material given per unit of body weight or the amount of the poison per unit volume of air respired. In some instances, it is critical to give the duration of time during which the poison was administered. Conveniently, the dose of a poison, whether actually administered by weight or by volume, is expressed in terms of units of weight.

Milligrams of poison per kilogram of body weight (mg/kg) is the usual form of expression. If especially large doses are involved, it may be convenient to use *grams per kilogram* (gm/kg). If the doses are especially small, the expressions *micrograms of poison per kilogram of body weight* (μg/kg) or even *nanograms per kilogram* (ng/kg) may be used.

Often it is more informative to convert volume measurements of a dose (such as volume of alcohol) to the comparable weight unit; ordinarily it is satisfactory to assume that liquids have a density of 1 and thus 1 ml (1 cu. c) represents 1,000 mg.

Body weights are now converted to kilograms, even if the original data are shown as pounds of body weight. Since Congress has ruled that the metric system will be the standard in the United States in a few years, there is little to be gained by continuing with the conventional American way of handling weights and measures, despite the severe problems that may arise from the conversion.

From time to time, no information is available for the weight of a person, who may have been poisoned. As a general guideline, it is suggested that the standard physiological man, woman, or child be used in these instances:

Standard physiological man weighs 70 kg.
Standard physiological woman weighs 50 kg.
Standard physiological child weighs 20 kg.

Poisons are not restricted to a single kind of material. All the following materials contain substances that are poisonous: drugs, food additives, preservatives, ores, dyes, detergents, lubricants, soaps, plastics, gases, household chemicals, industrial intermediates, and waste products from a wide variety of production processes.

How a Poison Acts

A poison, to have an effect on the human body, must first get into the body. There are numerous routes by which toxic materials can enter the body. First, the poison may be swallowed and then absorbed from the digestive tract, entering the bloodstream, from where it is distributed throughout the body. This route of entry is known as the *gastrointestinal route.*

Some poisons are readily absorbed directly through the unbroken skin. This route is called the *percutaneous route.* Many of the modern organic phosphate insecticides (which are chemical relatives of the military "nerve gases") pass through the skin easily; parathion is an example.

Many poisons can enter the body by inhalation in the form of a gas, vapor, aerosol, or fine dust. This is the *pulmonary route.*

Most poisons splashed into the eye are absorbed into the blood through the surface of the eye, the *perocular* or *ocular route.*

In biomedical experimentation, poisons are often injected into the body using a hypodermic needle and syringe. The injection may be made directly into a blood vessel, the *intravenous route.* Poisons may be injected just below the skin into the space between the muscles and the skin covering, the *subcutaneous route.* Injections directly into the mass of a muscle are *intramuscular.* At times the injection is through the belly wall and into the body cavity in the abdominal region, the *intraperitoneal route.* For special experiments, injections are made between the ribs directly into the chest cavity, the *intrathoracic route.*

It should be obvious that antidotes for poisons and drugs used in the treatment of poisoning can be administered via any one of the above routes.

At the Individual Body Cell

After the poison gets into the bloodstream, it must be transported to the organ or tissue where it causes an effect. In order to act, the poison must diffuse to the surface of cells with special receptor sites for that kind of poison molecule. Once the molecule of poison reaches the cell surface or membrane, it is absorbed or attached to the surface, where it is prepared for permeation of the cell membrane or passage through the membrane into the cell itself. Once the poison gets into the living body cell, it alters the metabolism (the sum total of all the chemical reactions going on in the cell) of that cell and in that way expresses itself as the biologically active chemical we classify as a poison.

A few very specialized poisons do not permeate the cell but remain absorbed to the surface of the cell, the cell membrane. There they exert their effect by changing the functional processes going on at and in the cell membrane.

Nevertheless, matters related to the permeability of the surface of the cell are of the first importance because most of the time, the membrane surrounding the cell is the physical structure that determines the rate at which the signs and symptoms of poisoning occur and the progress of the poisoning action.

Of course, the nature of the poison molecule has an important role in the activity of a chemical as a poison. For example, a smaller molecule generally has a more rapid action than a larger one. The electric charge on the poison molecule modifies the rate at which the poison can enter cells and thus the rate at which the poison can exert its effects. Solubility in fatty substances seems also to be associated with more rapid biological action of a poisonous chemical.

Mechanisms of Action

Virtually all poisons act in one of the following ways. Some inhibit the action of critical enzyme systems or alter the specific action of certain enzymes. An enzyme is a substance that acts as a catalyst (a facilitator of chemical reactions) in various biochemical processes in the body. An example of the enzyme-inhibiting poisons is parathion, which in the body is converted to paraoxon.

The latter is a powerful inhibitor of the action of cholinesterase, an enzyme important in the normal functioning of the human nervous system. Certain enzymes alter the molecular structure of key chemicals by various means. When these chemicals (some of them may be enzymes) are altered, even in a minor fashion, they no longer can serve their normal function in the body, and the process of which they are an integral part is disrupted.

Other poisons act to change the permeability of various membranes or barriers in the body. The result is, in effect, the "short-circuiting" of critical biochemical pathways.

The action of some poisons is what can be called mechanical. These are the corrosive types that burn and corrode tissues and destroy them in a gross fashion. A blow torch or a rasp or a gouge used appropriately would have the same result.

Modifiers of Toxic Action

There are a number of conditions that in general modify the action of a poisonous substance.

The amount of the material taken is important. The amount of a poison needed to be toxic is usually expressed in terms of the MLD or minimum lethal dose. This quantity is the smallest amount of the poisonous material usually deadly to an adult. It is interesting that an overdose of certain poisons may be nonlethal to the subject because vomiting is induced, which tends to rid the body of the poison. Oxalic acid, for example, if taken in excessive amounts, causes vomiting; this reaction prevents the poisonous action of the acid.

Habit may itself modify the action of a poison on the body. Tolerance is developed to some poisons. We know that individuals who have a habit of taking large amounts of alcohol or opium eventually show great tolerance for excessive amounts, even amounts that would have killed them before they developed the tolerance. There is also the cumulative effect of certain poisons. These toxic substances in small amounts seem to act to successively weaken the subject until the final dose need not be as heavy as an earlier dose.

Idiosyncracy is most important in evaluating the action of a poison. Certain people have a great susceptibility to various drugs. For example, a few individuals in any population can be poisoned readily by aspirin. One tablet of aspirin may have severe depressing action on the heart. Most individuals can take a significant amount of aspirin without any harmful effects, but those who have this idiosyncracy to the action of aspirin can be readily killed by ordinarily harmless levels of the poison.

Age influences the susceptibility of an individual to poison. In general, immature individuals are more susceptible than are adults. On the other hand, very old people tolerate many poisons quite poorly.

State of health is quite obviously a factor that modifies the reaction to a poison. Poisons in general are more potent in sick individuals than in healthy individuals; for example, persons who have nephritis or some inflammatory disease of the kidneys show dangerous responses to morphine and hyoscine. Individuals who have developed cirrhosis of the liver show a wide variety of dangerous responses to drugs, whereas healthy individuals given similar doses are unaffected by these drugs. Inflammation of the gut (enteritis) results in certain drugs such as arsenic having especially potent effects.

The route by which the poison gets into the body and the *rate* at which it enters the body both influence the biological action significantly. The route of entry may be through the skin (percutaneous) or by various other ways. The order of increasing effectiveness of a poison in terms of route of entry is as follows: percutaneous, followed by oral (by mouth), intramuscular, subcutaneous, and intravenous, while the most effective is inhalation.

A full stomach generally decreases the toxic action of a poison that enters the body by being swallowed. The dramatic effect known as the *crash concentration* caused by many poisons is characterized as follows: If a large amount is given quickly, the devastating effect is much greater than if that same amount of poison is given more slowly. In the latter instance, the natural detoxicating mechanisms of the body have a chance to destroy some of the poison before it can be effective. In the crash concentration, the detoxicating mechanisms of the body are completely overwhelmed and the adverse action of the drug occurs before the natural defenses of the body can be brought into play.

As an example of the different kinds of toxicity, Table 1-I gives the minimum lethal dose for a 160 pound man of various common poisons.

Table 1-I
MLD OF SOME COMMON POISONS
FOR A 160 POUND MAN

Arsenic	200 mg	Camphor	2 gm
Strychnine	100 mg	Chlorates	8 gm
Nicotine	60 mg	Mercuric chloride	0.5 gm
Aconitine	10 mg	Organic phosphates	15 mg
Chloral	5 gm	Phenol	15 ml
DDT	15 gm	Boric acid	10 gm
Barbiturates	1-6 gm	Cresol	8 gm
Formaldehyde	50 ml	Croton oil	1 ml
Whiskey	1 qt.	"1080," sodium fluoroacetate	
Cantharidin	30 mg		50 mg

Classification of Poisons

There are a number of ways that poisons can be classified for convenience of study. They may be classified according to the effects produced on the body, according to chemical or physical nature of the poisons themselves, by the analytical behavior, or by their origin.

Effects Produced on the Body

Under this category first are *corrosives*. These are poisons that are either acids or alkalies. They act to eat away or corrode tissues. The corrosive substances or corrosive poisons include irritant gases, caustic alkalies, corrosive inorganic acids, corrosive organic acids, and heavy metals.

Second are the *irritants*. Among the irritants are arsenic, iodine, and cantharides. These poisons irritate certain specific tissues of the body. For example, cantharides are made up of the dried ground-up parts of an insect. If ingested as part of food or drink, the material causes severe irritation and inflammation of the urinary passages of the body. It has been used illegally and mistakenly as an aphrodisiac, with the popular and dangerous belief that if given to a female in food or drink, it will cause sexual aggression on her part and thus make her receptive to the advances of a male. This does not occur; what does occur is that the cantharides cause vigorous irritation of the urinary passages and can cause inflammation severe enough to result in disability and even permanent damage to the person given this substance.

Next are the narcotics, such as alcohol, opium, and barbiturates. These poisons have a depressing effect on the body. When taken in large amounts, they depress the respiration and circulation, leading to unconsciousness and death.

ANOXIA. It is possible to look at these categories of poisoning based on the main pathological findings observed when the body of a victim is autopsied. Under these conditions, there is a group of poisons that cause death by anoxia or lack of oxygen. Some of these poisons combine with the hemoglobin in the blood and thus prevent oxygen from combining with the hemoglobin. These poisons may also render the hemoglobin inactive. In any event, anoxia results. Carbon monoxide and the nitrites are examples of this class of poison.

A second group of poisons that cause death by anoxia acts to paralyze the respiratory enzymes in the various cells of the body; a typical example of this category is the cyanides. There are poisons that destroy the blood-forming organs of the body; radioactive substances kill by destroying the blood-forming organs and thus bringing about anoxia. There are also substances that are called radiomimetic; these are substances that mimic the effect of radioactive materials and destroy the blood-forming organs.

PROTOPLASMIC POISONS. Another group of poisons seen at autopsy is what are known as the protoplasmic and parenchymatous poisons. These poisons are toxic to the cells of the body and to the capillaries in the blood system after they actually have been absorbed into the body. They also seem to possess a local irritating effect, which may be of less significance than the direct action on the cells and the capillaries. A common outcome of these poisons is a *pathological* condition known as fatty degeneration of many organs, such as the liver, kidneys, or some other key organ.

There is a tendency of poisons of this sort, because of their action on the capillaries, to cause hemorrhages. Among these poisons are phosphorus and carbon tetrachloride.

NERVOUS SYSTEM TOXICITY. Finally, there are poisons that have a selective toxicity to zero in on the nervous system. Among these poisons are the anesthetics, the hypnotic drugs, the narcotics, alcohol, some of the alkaloids, and some of the glycosides.

Chemical Nature

The chemical or physical nature of poisons themselves allows us to break them down into inorganic poisons, gaseous poisons, alkaloidal poisons, and nonalkaloidal poisons.

Analytical Behavior

The analytical behavior of those poisons is used as the method of classifying them, especially by laboratory technicians who want to isolate the various poisons for information to be given to prosecutors, police officers, and others.

First of all there are poisons that are *volatile*. These poisons tend to become vapors in steam when treated in an acid or in an alkaline solution. Other poisons are those that can be *extracted by ether* from an acid solution. The unknown material is acidified and then shaken with ether; certain poisons dissolve in ether and can be separated from all other poisons. There are poisonous materials that can be extracted by ether and similar solvents from an alkaline solution. Nearly all these ether-extractable poisons from alkaline solutions are themselves called alkaloids. Finally, there are the metals and the metalloids, which behave in a similar way with respect to various chemical analytical agents.

Classification by Origin

Many toxicologists not primarily concerned with analytical procedures classify poisons according to their origins. Many poisons are found in ordinary household chemical preparations, in preparations used to coat surfaces of useful devices and the like. Using this system of classification, one finds poisonous minerals, poisonous plants, industrial contaminants, pesticides, a variety of domestic materials, drugs, and even food and water.

Poisoning of Human Beings

The malicious use of poison against human beings is rare in the United States. Usually, when a poisoning occurs it is accidental. In the few cases of homicidal poisoning, the agent employed is usually a readily available poison such as a rodenticide or strychnine.

Human accidental poisonings, however, are still too common for us to take comfort. Most of the human poisonings that appear on a routine basis involve accidents to children. Children are inquisitive by nature. They are indiscriminate in their sampling of materials by mouth. It is essential that small children be treated as small children. Nothing harmful should be left within their reach.

General Signs of Poisoning

There are a number of biological reactions that result when a human being is exposed to a poisonous substance. The nature of these reactions or signs is sometimes helpful in identifying a specific poison or at least a special class of poisons. Among the signs of poisoning are the following.

VOMITING. Vomiting usually occurs after the following poisons are taken into the human body by mouth: arsenic, antimony, aconite, acids, alkalies, colchicine, cantharides, veratrum, phosphorus, mercury, iodine, and poisonous foods in general. Certain diseases also induce vomiting and can confuse this sign of poisoning, as can gastrointestinal upsets of various kinds. Vomiting is also observed in diseases such as uremia, cholera, and acidosis.

CONVULSIONS. Mild and even violent convulsions are observed after poisoning by a variety of chemical agents. Convulsions are seen after poisoning with strychnine, organic phosphates, camphor, cyanides, and aspidium. Because organic phosphates are used so widely on the farm, in the home, and in places of business to control and eradicate insect pests, these compounds are reasonably suspected when convulsions are observed in an individual who may have been exposed to a poison. There are a number of diseases that also cause convulsions in man; Among these are uremia, tetanus (lockjaw), meningitis, and epilepsy.

COMA. A variety of poisons result in the victim becoming unconscious and unresponsive to stimuli. Among the poisons that induce coma in the victim are opium and its derivatives, chloral, veronal, barbiturates, carbon monoxide, carbon dioxide, atropine, hyoscine, phenols, and alcohol. Alcohol poisoning to the point of coma is becoming more common than it used to be. A number of natural diseases are known to induce coma in individuals afflicted. Among these diseases are uremia, hemorrhage, and brain injury. Because brain injury is associated with coma in many instances, it is essential that victims found in a comatose state be handled with great care to avoid the possibility of aggravating a brain injury that might exist.

DILATION OF PUPIL OF THE EYE. Some poisons cause the pupil of the eye to dilate; among these poisons are belladonna, cocaine, nicotine, organic phosphates, and stramonium. Individuals who are suspected of being under the influence of a poison should be examined quickly to ascertain whether there is dilation of the pupils or not. There is a group of diseases or injuries that also results in dilation of the pupils of the eyes. These are nervous diseases that affect the optic nerve or the ocular motor nerve. In many instances of these diseases, the dilation of the pupil in each eye may be different in degree.

CONTRACTION OF PUPIL OF THE EYE. There are also poisons that cause the pupil of the eye to contract. In sufficient doses, some of these poisons result in pupils that are so contracted as to give a pinpoint appearance. Among these poisons are opium derivatives, the anticholinesterases (among these are the organic phosphate insecticides), pilocarpine, and muscarine. There are various nervous disabilities that can also result in contraction of the pupils of the eyes. In many instances, the contraction of the pupils is unequal.

There have been homicides in which morphine (which contracts the pupils) has been mixed with atropine (which dilates the pupils) and the mixture then was given to the victim. These drugs in the proper proportion acted against one another (were antagonistic) with the end result that the pupillary response was erased and the pupils in the poisoned subject looked to be of normal diameter. Adequate toxicological analyses of the body fluids in these victims would of course reveal the presence of the two drugs.

GENERAL AND PARTIAL PARALYSIS. A number of toxic agents cause a general paralysis or a partial paralysis in the individual poisoned. Such poisons include cyanides, carbon monoxide and carbon dioxide, and botulism. The latter is probably the most potent poison known to man. It is produced by a species of bacteria found in foods. Ordinarily, one does not run into botulism poisoning apart from accidental eating of inadequately canned foods. The pure poison is not available other than in restricted amounts to research institutions. Certain diseases such as brain tumors and meningitis also cause general or partial paralysis.

SLOWED RESPIRATION. Poisons such as carbon monoxide and opium serve to depress the rate of respiration. Individuals under the influence of these poisons show a significantly decreased rate of breathing. Similar slowed down respiration is seen in such diseases as uremia or in accidents that result in compression of the brain.

INCREASED RESPIRATION. Other poisons bring about an increased rate of respiration. Among these poisons are atropine, carbon dioxide, and cocaine. There are also natural diseases that bring about increased respiration; for example, lesions of the medulla, a portion of the brain, are known to cause rapid respiration.

DYSPNEA. Difficulty in breathing or labored breathing is caused by strychnine, organic phosphates, cyanides, and carbon monoxide. There are also diseases that bring on this labored breathing, among them are cardiac and respiratory diseases generally, lesions of the vague nerve, and lesions of the medulla oblongata.

CYANOSIS. After poisoning with certain chemicals, the individual becomes cyanotic, that is, the skin takes on a bluish tinge. Red portions of the body such as the lips and the beds of the fingernails, instead of having a healthy red color, show a sickly bluish tinge. Among poisons that cause this cyanotic response are opium, acetanilid, aniline, and nitrobenzene. There are certain diseases that also bring on cyanosis, generally diseases of the circulatory system or the respiratory system.

The presence of cyanosis is a positive indication of some condition that prevents the arrival of adequate oxygen to the blood and tissues of the body. The absence of cyanosis cannot be interpreted as evidence that a specific poison or disease is not present. For example, cyanosis frequently accompanies poisoning with curare; it can be a positive sign that curare is a possible poisoning agent. But the absence of cyanosis in no way can be used as evidence that curare poisoning has not occurred. A number of factors can mask the development of cyanosis. Thus the generalized bluishness of the skin can be indicative of certain poisons; its absence cannot be indicative of the absence of these poisons.

Change in Urine Following Poisoning

Most poisons taken into the body are eventually eliminated through the urine. Consequently, the reactions of urine are useful in arriving at some indication of what poison an individual may have been subjected to. It is not maintained that examination of the urine is adequate to diagnose precisely what poison is harming an individual. However, a quick indication or suggestion of what poison might be causing trouble may be obtained from a simple test of the urine of the victim. Table 1-II should be useful in clarifying this point.

Acute and Chronic Toxicity

ACUTE POISONING. Poisons may act acutely or chronically. Acute poisoning results from a comparatively large dose of a poison given in a very short period of time. The action is fairly rapid. There is no buildup of the poison over a long period of time; death or disability results within a matter of minutes, hours, or at most a day. Most homicidal poisonings are the result of an acute dose of a poison. Similarly, most suicidal poisonings are the result of the victim taking a large dose of some toxic material at a single time and then expiring or becoming acutely ill in a short period of time.

CHRONIC POISONING. On the other hand, many environmental

Table 1-II

THE QUALITATIVE REACTION OF URINE IN HUMAN BEINGS TO
VARIOUS POISONS

Reaction	Poisons
1. Very acid	1. Acids, metallic salts
2. Very alkaline	2. Alkalies, salts of organic acids, except oxalic
3. Violet color	3. Turpentine, ethereal oils
4. Garlic odor	4. Tellurium, compounds of tellurium
5. Ammonia odor	5. Strong bases
6. Yellow to deep red	6. Picrates, picric acid, acriflavin, selenium
7. Red after addition of sodium hydroxide	7. Senna leaves, phenolphthalein, cascara sagrada, antipyrin
8. Port-wine color	8. Sulfonal, chronic lead
9. Conjugated sulfates	9. Phenol, cresol, lysol®, acetanilid phenacetin
10. Leucin and tyrosin	10. Phosphorus
11. Drop in eye of cat dilates pupil	11. Atropine, hyposcyamine, scopolamine, cocaine
12. Drop causes tetantus in frog or small mouse	12. Strychnine
13. Garlic odor after adding to culture of *Penicillium brevicaule*	13. All arsenic compounds except triphenarsines; selenium and tellurium compounds

poisons including poisonings related to one's job are termed
chronic. Chronic poisonings usually result from the repeated or
constant exposure of an individual to relatively small amounts of
poison at any given time. It is the long-term or repeated exposure
that builds up a poisoning level that eventually either kills or
disables the individual.

TESTING POISONS. The testing of poisons for their acute action
is relatively simple. Uncomplicated tests of the LD_{50} can be set up
with a minimum of effort and expense. On the other hand,
chronic toxicity testing is complicated, time-consuming, and ex-
pensive. Gaddum (1953) discussed at length the requirements,
biological and mathematical, for carrying out toxicity testing.

How Much Material for Forensic Chemical Analysis?

In many instances, a law enforcement officer is required to
attend the postmortem examination of the poisoned victim. He is

there to observe, to answer questions of the pathologist, and to accept items of physical evidence that the pathologist may wish to turn over to the police. The law enforcement officer can also be a valuable resource to the pathologist in answering a variety of questions. Among these questions are how much tissue or how much body fluid is needed to carry out a satisfactory toxicological examination. This section attempts to answer briefly and reasonably this particular question.

URINE. All the urine that can be obtained from the bladder of the deceased should be collected in a clean bottle, sealed, and brought to the toxicologist.

STOMACH CONTENTS. In poisoning cases, all the stomach contents and all the intestinal contents should be preserved. The easiest way to preserve the stomach contents is to have the pathologist tie off the stomach at each end. In effect, then, the contents are tied into a bag consisting of the stomach wall. The stomach with the contents is then put into a large plastic evidence bag or into a large jar without preservative or any other foreign material. In that form, it is delivered to the toxicologist. The intestinal contents can be stripped into a large chemically clean jar and all the material taken to the toxicologist.

BLOOD. No less than 100 ml of blood should be made available.

BRAIN AND LIVER. Brain and liver also should be tested for poisons. At least 500 grams of the tissue should be put into a clean plastic bag or a chemically clean jar with a tight lid. If at all possible, one-half of the brain, either the right or the left half, is desirable. A large lobe of the liver is also desirable. But in any event, no less than 500 gm should be taken.

OTHER TISSUES. Samples of bone, muscle, and body fat should be at least 200 grams each. Any less makes it difficult for the toxicologist if he must do repeat tests. One whole kidney should be taken for chemical analysis. In children who are poisoned, it is desirable that both kidneys be removed from the body and made available to the toxicologist.

BILE. Bile quite often contains drugs and poisons that have been taken into the body. The bile then is funneled into the intestine, where these materials can be eliminated. Consequently, samples of bile should be taken. The best way is to tie off the gall bladder securely and remove it entirely from the body, much as the stomach was removed. It is put into a clean plastic evidence bag or into a chemically clean jar with a secure lid. There really is not much point trying to take a small amount of bile out of the gall bladder when it is much simpler to remove the entire gall bladder after tying it off so that none of the bile spills out.

EYE FLUID. In some cases in which alcohol is a poison of concern, there may be a problem of contamination of the blood. It is therefore strongly desirable that eye fluid be removed at the time of the autopsy and put into chemically clean vials. The fluid in the eye reflects quite precisely the alcohol content of the blood. Moreover, the fluid in the eye is not subject to contamination as readily as is the blood. Consequently, it is strongly suggested that eye fluid be taken whenever a toxicological examination is necessary.

If there is any doubt at the time of autopsy whether a given tissue or fluid should be removed and preserved for analysis, the simple answer is when in doubt, take it out. If the material is not needed, it then can be disposed of according to the laws of the particular state in question. If the material is needed, it sometimes can be critical. Once the body is embalmed, the removal of tissues for chemical analysis may be an exercise in futility. It is much better to take more than is needed when the tissues are available than to attempt to rectify an oversight at a later date.

ACCIDENTAL POISONINGS. When a poisoning incident is investigated, the probability that it is accidental is high. Less probably is it suicidal. Least probable of all is homicidal poisoning. This assertion does not mean that murder by poison never occurs; it means only that poison in this day and age in the United States is a rarely used weapon of the murderer.

Of all accidental poisonings recorded nationally, 65 percent of them occur in children who are five years old or younger, 6 percent occur in children between five and fourteen years of age, and 21 percent are found in persons over fifteen years of age. About 7 percent of the poisonings happen to persons whose age is unknown for some reason or other.

Table 1-III shows the distribution of accidental poisonings by toxicant (poisonous chemical involved) for the various age-groups. Medicines are by far the agents most often causing accidental poisonings. Despite concern for poisons such as carbon monoxide, the table shows that toxic gases and vapors are responsible for an insignificant (statistically) number of accidental poisonings.

Table 1-III

MOST COMMON CHEMICAL AGENTS CAUSING ACCIDENTAL POISONINGS

Toxicant	Age-Groups				
	Less than 5 years	5 to 14	Over 14	Unknown	All Ages
Medicines	45	47	80	40	52
Aspirin	8	7	6	3	7
Other internal	29	36	72	31	39
External	8	4	3	6	7
Cleaning and polishing agents	16	8	4	15	13
Petroleum products	4	4	2	4	4
Cosmetics	8	2	0.6	4	6
Pesticides	5	5	2	9	5
Turpentine, paints, etc.	6	4	1	5	5
Plants	5	8	1	6	4
Gases and vapors	0.2	2	2	3	0.8
Miscellaneous	8	17	4	13	8
Unknown	0.9	2	4	1	2

*Values are given in percentages of total poisonings in each age-group based on data from the National Clearing House for Poison Information Centers. *See also* Haggerty (1975).

The second group of toxicants of importance in accidental poisonings is preparations used for cleaning and polishing. Nevertheless, the careful control of medicines in the home and elsewhere would have the greatest impact on curtailing accidental poisonings in the United States. Some of the accidental poisonings result in death to the victims. The causative agents in fatal poisonings are shown in Table 1-IV.

Of all the drug deaths that are accidental, 50 percent of them in children less than five years old apparently are caused by sali-

Table 1-IV
CHEMICALS CAUSING DEATH IN ACCIDENTAL POISONINGS*

Toxicant	Less than 5 Years Old	Total Deaths
Medicines		
Salicylates and pain killers	28	19
Sedatives	4	24
Psychotherapeutic drugs	5	4
Other	20	16
TOTAL DRUGS	57	63
Household products		
Alcohol	0.4	7
Petroleum and solvents	12	2
Pesticides	10	2
Heavy metals	7	1
Other	13	25
TOTAL NONDRUGS	43	37

*Values are given in percentages of total deaths by age for all poisoning deaths.

cylates (aspirin) and other pain killers. Only 31 percent of the total of accidental drug deaths (for all ages) are so caused. Sedatives and hypnotics account for 6 percent of the medicine-caused deaths in those five years of age or younger but account for 38 percent of all the medicine-caused deaths. Psychotherapeutic drugs cause 9 percent of the drug deaths in those five years old or younger and 6 percent of all drug deaths. An assortment of "other" medicines accounts for 36 percent of all the medicine-related accidental poisonings (Table 1-IV).

For household products, the percentage of deaths from the various items by age-group as compared to the total deaths from these "home chemicals" is given in Table 1-V.

Table 1-V
DEATHS FROM HOUSEHOLD PRODUCTS*

	Less than 5 Years Old	Total
Alcohol	1	18
Petroleum and solvents	28	6
Pesticides	24	5
Heavy metals	17	4
Other	30	67

*Values are given in percentages of age-groups.

For the young child, pesticides and petrochemicals pose the greatest threat to life among the usual household chemicals. Among all such deaths, however, there is a large unknown area of assorted chemicals ("Other" in Table 1-V) that are death dealing. Alcohol is also not an inconsiderable factor in accidental deaths across the board caused by chemicals.

Some Factors that Influence Poisoning Action

There are a number of factors that modify the poisoning action of a given substance. Because of these influencing factors, often a specific case of poisoning may be confusing, especially to the nonexpert.

Slight modifications in an experimental design can change in a drastic fashion the response of an animal or some other system to the same poisonous substance. Indeed, one finds that in the analysis for different poisons, there are confusing and confounding factors that can becloud the results of an analytical procedure.

For example, the composition of a particular sample collected for analysis can show false results if one is not extremely careful in the analytical procedures. Moreover, sometimes a poison is dissolved in some liquid. The liquid itself may have a biological effect that can confuse the poisoning pattern.

There is a fundamental principle in toxicology known as *synergism,* well-known but often ignored. It might be explained as follows: If two poisonous substances are given simultaneously in a mixture to a target organism such as man, these poisons may act together in an additive way. In other words, poison A plus poison B will give essentially the effect equal to the arithmetic sum of the two poisons. Such poisons act additively. However, frequently when two poisons of this sort are administered simultaneously, the total effect is greater than the arithmetic sum of the individual actions. This is like saying that 1 plus 2 does not equal 3, rather 1 plus 2 equals 6. In this type of action, the poisons are *synergistic;* they act together to give an effect greater than the simple combined effects of the two poisons.

Another aspect of poisons given together is that they may act *antagonistically.* In other words, if the two poisonous substances are given together, the total effect may be less than one would expect from simple addition of the individual effects.   The substances act against one another, as it were.

The actual mixture administered as a poison can modify the absorption of the poison; it can modify its availability once it gets into the body.   A discussion of the factors that can influence the toxicity of a given poison follows.

THE POISON ITSELF.   There are factors in toxicity that are related to *the poison itself.*   These include the chemical composition; the acidity or the alkalinity of the mixture has an effect. There are certain physical characteristics such as the *size of the particle* of the individual poison or whether it is administered in powder form, for example, that make a difference.   If impurities or other contaminating materials are present, the toxic action may be modified.   The *shelf life* of the poison is important   Some poisons are stable, others tend to break down during storage.   Consequently, the stability and the characteristics on the shelf of the toxic agent are important.   The *solubility* of the poison in body fluids is a factor.   If a poison is not readily dissolved in the various body fluids, it will not be as rapidly poisonous as a substance that is quickly and readily dissolved.   The choice of the solvent, or what is sometimes called the *vehicle,* can modify the action of a poison.   There are a number of *other factors* such as coating agents, coloring agents, flavoring agents, preservatives and so on that can affect how a poison acts.

EXPOSURE TO THE POISON.   There are factors that are related to the exposure, including the *actual dose.*   If the dose of poison is too small, the bodily defense mechanisms can take over, and the individual does not show any serious toxic responses.   The *concentration* of a poison is important.   For example, carbon monoxide in air is relatively harmless as long as it does not reach a certain level.   After the concentration gets above a certain minimal level, trouble can result.   The *volume* of the material that gets into the body is also important.   Poisons get into the body through a number of *routes:*   by ingestion, through the skin, through the eye, or absorbed in the lungs.   The route by which the poison gets into the body is important in the overall toxic effect the poison may have.

The *rate* at which poison is administered is also important. For example, a person can breathe in a large amount of carbon monoxide spread over a long period of time without showing any adverse effects. If that total amount of carbon monoxide were breathed into the body in a shorter period of time, the person might be killed. Consequently, both *route* and *rate* of entry of a poison into the body have profound influence on the toxicity.

Some poisons tend to pile up, as it were; the duration of exposure to a poison and the frequency of exposure may also modify the poisonous action. Finally, there is another action that has only recently come into interest—the time at which the poison gets into the body. This aspect might be called the *diurnal* or *seasonal* aspect of exposure to a poison. It is now known that there are different times of the day at which poisons getting into the human body have a greater effect than other times of the day. Studies with experimental animals have shown that there may be more serious effects if poisons are taken during the later afternoon than if they are taken into the body during the morning. Poisons that are taken into the body during daylight may act differently than when they are taken during the nighttime hours. There are also seasonal variations and even yearly modifications in susceptibility to poisons. It is important, therefore, to understand that these kinds of environmental factors can and do change the toxic effect of poisons.

THE VICTIM. Obviously there are factors peculiar to the subject or victim. Certain *genetic characters* may make a person more susceptible to a given poison or less susceptible. We are at the moment pitifully ignorant of the total implications of genetics in the response of individuals to poisons. Some individuals are more sensitive to certain poisons than are others; this sensitivity seems to be related to what is called the *immunologic status* of the individual. *Nutritional factors* are also important. If a person is in a poor state of nutrition, he is probably more susceptible to poisons than a person who is adequately fed. The status of the endocrine system or the *hormonal balance* of the body also is important. Women who are pregnant have certain susceptibilities to poisons that the nonpregnant woman does not. On the other hand, pregnant women show certain strong resistances to some toxic substances, whereas in their nonpregnant condition, they would be more susceptible.

Age, sex, body weight, and sexual maturity all influence the effect of poison on the body. For example, DDT given to newborn mice must be given in enormous doses to have the same effect as a dose 100 times smaller would have in an adult mouse. There are certain types of diseases or disabilities of various organ systems that render some people more susceptible to certain poisons than others.

CONDITIONS SURROUNDING THE VICTIM. Activity, crowding, the presence of other people, and so on may all have an effect on the response to a poison. Last but not least are *environmental factors* that surround the subject or victim. Certain poisons are influenced by the temperature or the humidity in which a person finds himself. Atropine, for example, has a much greater adverse effect in a desert situation than in a cool, moist climate.

The effect of *barometric pressure* is well-known. For example, in Colorado on Sunday afternoons, it is not uncommon for parties in automobiles going over the high mountain passes to end up with one or two passengers, especially children, in a semicomatose state as a result of carbon monoxide getting into the automobile at these very high altitudes (low barometric pressure). A similar concentration of carbon monoxide at sea level would have little or no effect. A whole variety of atmospheric conditions may influence the effect of poisons, including light, heat, and so on. Noise also has an effect, as well as social factors and a variety of unknown chemical factors.

Relative Toxicities

In discussing toxic materials, it is important to know the actual amount of material that gets into a man and the effect that is called *toxic, very toxic,* or *super toxic.*

In talking about the human being as the target of a poison, a standard reference is made in the biomedical sciences to the 70 kg male (150 pound man). However, all men do not weigh 150 pounds. For the sake of having some kind of a standard "reference man," toxicologists use, arbitrarily if you will, a man weighing 70 kg or 150 pounds.

The relative toxicities of various poisonous agents then are referred to the standard man. A convenient way of comparing the toxicities of different substances is to use a toxicity ratio starting from Number 1 (which would include substances that are practically nonpoisonous) to Number 6 (substances that could be called *super toxic*). Table 1-VI illustrates such a scale of relative toxicities (Hodge and Sterner, 1949; Gleason et al., 1969).

Table 1-VI
SCALE OF RELATIVE TOXICITIES

Number	Killing Dose	Definition
1	15 gm/kg; @ 1 qt. or more	Nontoxic
2	5-15 gm/kg.; @ 1 pt. to 1 qt.	Slightly toxic
3	0.5-5 gm/kg; @ 1 oz. to 1 pt. or 1 lb.	Moderately toxic
4	50-500 mg/kg; 1 tsp. to 1 oz.	Very toxic
5	5-50 mg/kg; 7 drops to 1 tsp.	Extremely toxic
6	5 mg/kg or less; a mere taste to @ 7 drops	Super toxic

There is a wide variety of substances that are toxic to man in various levels of potency. The toxicologist must be familiar with substances in all these categories. As new substances become available, he is challenged to understand them and their toxic properties.

Circulation Time of Blood. Circulation time is the rapidity with which a volume of blood moves from one part of the body to another. How fast a poison acts on a human being depends in part upon how rapidly the toxic agent moves from the point of entry to the target organ or tissue where the effects occur.

Table 1-VII gives an idea of the circulation time between several points in the human body.

Human Blood Volume and Water Content of Body. Any poison taken into the body is diluted by the total amount of blood

Table 1-VII

CIRCULATION TIME OF BLOOD

Distance	Average Time in Seconds	Range in Seconds
From arm to foot	43	20-55
Arm to hand on opposite side	17	
Arm to lungs	—	3-8
Arm to brain	—	6-12

and body water in that body. The average total blood volume of man is 65 to 70 ml/kg of body weight. The "standard" 70 kg man has between 4550 and 4900 ml of blood (4.6 to 4.9 liters; 9.7 to 10.4 pints).

The total body water in man is proportionately greater in thin persons than in fat persons. In infants, water accounts for about 80 percent of their body weight. In adults, water accounts for about 66 to 75 percent of the body weight.

It is possible to estimate the total amount of alcohol, drug, or poison in the human body if the amount in a given organ is known:

$$\text{Total in male body} = \frac{0.7 \text{ weight of body} \times \text{weight of chemical found}}{\text{Weight of organ tested}}$$

The number 0.7 is a factor for expressing the proportion of chemical agent (poison) in the body to that in the tissues. The factor is about 0.7 for men, about 0.5 to 0.6 for women.

ORGAN WEIGHT AS PERCENTAGE OF BODY WEIGHT. The composition of the average male human body is relatively constant. The various organs each make up a fixed percentage of the total weight of the body (Simpson, 1967). Table 1-VIII is useful in summarizing the percentages of the total body weight accounted for by the respective organs listed.

Knowing the weight of a single organ, one may estimate from this table the total body weight; knowing the body weight, the weight of a given organ may be estimated.

Table 1-VIII

ORGAN WEIGHT AS PERCENTAGE OF BODY WEIGHT

Organ	Percent of Total Body Weight
Fat	14
Muscles	43
Bones, including marrow	14
Blood	8
Empty digestive tract	3
Lungs	1
Liver	2
Both kidneys	0.43
Spleen	0.2
Brain	2
Spinal cord	0.04
Eyes	0.04
Skin	3
Heart	0.43
Teeth	0.03
Other organs together	9

Chapter 2

RECOGNITION OF POISONING

Some Signs and Symptoms of the
Absorption of Small Amounts of Toxic Chemicals

THE INFORMATION AVAILABLE on the action of poisons in man ordinarily comes from extrapolation of the results obtained in animal experiments, the study of accidental poisonings, and reports from departments of industrial medicine in universities and industry. "The best source of information on the effects of foreign chemicals upon health is industrial medical reports" (Foulger, 1959).

Despite the fact that analytical chemistry has become remarkably sophisticated in the identification of poisonous substances in the human body, there are still limitations to the information that can be obtained quickly from the analytical chemist. Measurement of various compounds in urine samples reveals information of importance concerning the uptake of heavy metals. The value of urine analysis for many organic compounds is questionable. Many organic compounds are broken down in the body, and the breakdown products accumulate in the urine. The time during which the accumulation occurs is not always precise; consequently the measured concentration in the urine at any moment probably is a reflection of the accumulated result of an unknown period of exposure.

Individuals who accumulate small amounts of toxic chemicals ordinarily show a pattern of nonspecific signs and symptoms long before analytical data reveal that borderline poisoning is occurring. According to Foulger (1959), the signs and symptoms are "headache, nausea, dizziness, discomfort in the epigastrium, gastroin-

36

testinal upsets, poor appetite, excessive fatigue." Foulger further points out that a study of any book on toxicology reveals how this widespread group of symptoms may serve as early warnings of exposure to a chemical that has invaded the body by inhalation, absorption through the skin, or swallowing. These signs and symptoms seem to be the same despite the route by which the offending chemical entered the body.

How Do These Various Responses Occur?

HEADACHE. Headache ordinarily results from the dilation of blood vessels in or near the head region; pulling on these blood vessels as a result of muscle tension may also result in headache. Headache seems to be especially related to poisoning agents such as nitrites or histamine; these agents dilate the blood vessels in the brain area. Headache is also brought about by chemical agents that cause a sudden increase in the blood pressure in the body. Headache is not infrequently accompanied by nausea.

LOSS OF APPETITE. This response is sometimes referred to by medical personnel as *anorexia*. The control of appetite is located in the brain. How much of the appetite sense depends upon secretions from the stomach or from changes in the motility of the gastrointestinal tract is not clear. What is clear is that pain, fright, grief, and a variety of strong emotions result in the constriction of blood vessels in the wall of the stomach; there is a reduction in the contraction of muscles making up the stomach wall; there is a decrease in the secretion of hydrochloric acid into the stomach cavity. Drugs such as amphetamine reduce the appetite temporarily in concentrations that have no effect on the contractions of the stomach wall.

DIZZINESS. Dizziness has been defined as a disruption of the sense of one's relationship to space. It is also referred to as giddiness. There is a feeling of unsteadiness with a sensation of movement inside the head. Dizziness often is a sign that fainting will occur. In some instances it is caused by reduction of the oxygen supply to the brain.

The pattern of signs and symptoms indicated above often obtains in conditions that are known to involve a decrease of oxygen supply to the brain. Casual observations have indicated that the inhalation of oxygen for a short time may decrease the headache resulting from exposure to poisonous chemicals. The mechanism is not clear. What does seem clear is that "the production of these symptoms by reduction in oxygen supply and their frequent disappearance on administration of oxygen strongly suggests that fundamental oxidative mechanisms are involved" (Foulger, 1959). The circulation to the brain has effective regional control so that these symptoms can result from a localized decrease in oxygen content and not necessarily from an overall decrease in the oxygen available to the brain.

The symptoms that accompany the uptake by the human body of toxic chemicals are the same that are seen during acute infectious diseases. When these symptoms result from infection, ordinarily there is a fever. Frequently, these symptoms occur after the absorption of poisonous chemicals without any indication of fever. Usually the symptoms disappear rapidly when the victim is removed from the source of the toxic foreign chemical.

On the other hand, if an infectious disease is responsible, the symptoms persist as long as the invading organism is alive and functioning. The organism then serves as a constant source of some kind of toxic chemical that it produces and introduces into the body.

One of the most surprising observations in poisoning by toxic chemicals is the rapidity with which the fatigue and other adverse symptoms disappear when the exposure to these chemicals is eliminated. In some instances, the relief may occur within hours. In other instances, it may take a day or two. Usually the relief from adverse responses occurs much more rapidly than is observed after an infectious disease has been conquered by the body.

Police Implications

For the law enforcement officer, these signs and symptoms may be useful if he has reason to suspect that he is faced with a case of poisoning by some toxic chemical. In view of the fact that police officers are called in all sorts of emergencies, it might be well to keep these signs and symptoms in mind. Industrial firms, chemical laboratories, testing laboratories, a variety of machine shops, and other business activities can be the source of poisonous chemicals. Indeed, the patrolman's automobile can readily be the source of toxic chemicals. Carbon monoxide and other chemicals can seep into a patrol car, bringing on some of these signs and symptoms. Pesticides and cleaning agents can also produce vapors that cause this general complex of symptoms.

The important point to remember is that should such a complex of symptoms affect the law enforcement officer or be present in individuals located where he has been called for some purpose, it might be wise to call for medical aid as quickly as possible. As much detail as possible should be recorded with respect to the complaints of the individuals, sketches of the scene, and any possible sources of foreign chemicals. Then medical support should be called upon. Whatever that medical support unit is should be clearly informed of the observations made at the scene by the officer. Once this aspect has been carried out, then competent medical personnel should insure adequate treatment and prevention of further exposure. The officer's role is not one of an industrial hygienist. His role after getting competent medical support is to record all the facts and information he can gather in the event that criminal or civil litigation might evolve from the case he has been asked to investigate.

EVIDENCE IN POISONING CASES. The collection of physical evidence in connection with suspected crimes of poisoning is a critical operation (Fox and Cunningham, 1973). Poisoning cases usually pose difficult problems for the detectives investigating the case and for the coroner or medical examiner. Numerous poisons cause signs and symptoms that imitate a variety of diseases caused by other agents. This fact can confuse the issue and make it hard to decide whether a crime has actually been perpetrated. It is the best policy, should there be reason to suspect a poisoning, to carry out the investigation as if a homicide did occur. It may be that the investigation will reveal that the death was suicidal or accidental. Indeed, the only time one can discard the possibility of homicide is when accident, suicide, or natural causes have been established.

In recent years, the use of poisons in homicides has been severely limited. There are a number of reasons for this situation. In many instances, the selection of a poison is such that the victim is warned. Moreover, modern laboratory instrumentation and procedures are capable of detecting virtually any poison that can be used. Thus, a proper laboratory workup can, in most cases, uncover a homicide due to poison. Criminals who are informed about poisons and use them in an educated manner have a wide range of possibilities for carrying out their homicidal intent. As Fox and Cunningham (1973) point out: "To further compound the problem, suicides and accidental deaths by poisoning are sometimes very difficult to distinguish from a homicide."

ACCIDENTAL DEATHS. Accidental deaths due to poisoning can be confusing because of the interaction of several poisons in a synergistic way. If alcohol is drunk with certain kinds of medicines, an accidental death can result from failure of respiration. This interaction of drugs is sometimes used suicidally. An example of this sort of interaction is the drinking of alcohol after taking a dose of amphetamines. The amphetamines stimulate the respiration and circulation in the body. When alcohol is then drunk, the usual depressant reaction to alcohol does not occur, and the victim can readily drink a killing dose of alcohol before he passes out, as he ordinarily would without the amphetamines. "Accidental deaths due to poisoning may result from occupational hazards, carelessness in taking medicine, and improper installation or maintenance of machinery or equipment" (Fox and Cunningham, 1973).

IMPORTANCE OF SIGNS. It is important for the police officer investigating a poisoning incident to recognize that the signs and symptoms of a particular poison are identical whether one is faced with a homicide, a suicide, or an accident. The officer investigating the scene of the incident should ascertain whether the victim vomited and whether convulsions, diarrhea, or paralysis occurred. If such information is available, one should record whether the victim's breathing was slow or rapid and whether the pupils of the eye were contracted or dilated. Are there any changes in skin color? Did the victim complain of difficulty in swallowing just before his death? These characteristics are general indications of a systemic poisoning. In and of themselves they are not proof that poisoning occurred, but they are important observations to be used in connection with other evidence.

It is critical that any witness who had observed the victim just before he died be carefully interrogated. That person is an outstanding source of information concerning the signs and symptoms of poisoning. Should there be no such witness available, then the case rests heavily on whatever physical evidence is available at the scene of the crime.

The police investigator assigned to a poisoning case should prepare a detailed history of the activities of the victim during the three days preceding death. Included in this history should be a clarification of what medicines were taken and when they were taken. What was the last meal, when was it taken, and where was it eaten? Any medical history available could reveal information of great importance in the case.

THE TOXICOLOGIST. Obviously, materials of various sorts will be sent to the toxicologist for analysis. The toxicologist is the scientific specialist who is charged with the identification and recognition of poisons. He is an expert in the physiological effects of poisons on human beings and animals, and he also is familiar with the antidotes for various poisons. Most crime laboratories have some form of toxicological capability. The amount and quality of such support varies greatly from one crime laboratory to another. If a given crime laboratory has a limited toxicological capability, it should not frustrate the investigative efforts of the police. A full toxicological examination can be insured by making use of a combination of laboratories such as the local hospital, the laboratory of the coroner or medical examiner, and laboratories that may be available in nearby educational institutions. State crime laboratories usually keep a list of various local facilities that can provide toxicological services. These crime laboratories can suggest which local laboratory could be used for a given poison test.

POISON CONTAINERS. Should the officer investigating a possible poisoning come to the conclusion that the poison was taken accidentally, a careful search must be made for the container. Ordinarily, if the poisoning is suicidal or accidental, the container will probably be fairly close to the victim. The container may be empty, but should be checked carefully for fingerprints nevertheless. After that, it is wrapped carefully and sent to the analytical laboratory.

Every object that could be remotely connected to the case should be collected as potential evidence. Unwashed dishes, glassware, flatware, the contents of wastebaskets, envelopes, and containers of medicine all should be collected, marked, and forwarded for analysis. It is important that the items collected be individually marked and sealed and that the chain of custody of this evidence be unbroken.

Poisoned Animals. Now and then the police are asked to investigate the poisoning of a dog or some other animal. If a dog is found dead for unexplained reasons, it is safe to assume that a poisoning occurred. However, dogs and other animals sometimes die rapidly as the result of a potent disease caused by bacteria. Animals that are allowed to run wild, notably in the spring of the year, frequently die rapidly of natural disease. Sometimes wild animals die during the winter and then freeze. When the body thaws in the spring, the tissue of the thawed animal provides an excellent culture system for the growth of bacteria. Should this meat then be eaten by a dog, there are some kinds of microorganisms that can kill a dog, the symptoms rather closely resembling poisoning by strychnine. Veterinarians can provide valuable help in the investigation of animal poisonings.

Alcohol. Alcohol should be considered as a significant factor during the investigation of virtually any violent incident. "Beverage alcohol becomes important clue material in an attempt to link a poisoning case with alcoholic drink. There is usually good reason to suspect that alcohol may have been the medium for a poisoning because it can serve as a good solvent, and frequently a taste cover, for many kinds of poisonous substances. Alcohol can itself be poisonous (isopropyl or rubbing alcohol, for example). The investigator should not overlook the possible poisonous effect of beverage alcohol when taken with certain drugs or simply in sufficient quantity; however, this type of use is normally not crime connected" (Fox and Cunningham, 1973).

A number of years ago, an interesting case revolved around the wife of a scientist drinking a martini made with wood alcohol. The woman took several days to die, and a combination of physical signs and symptoms plus chemical analyses demonstrated beyond doubt that she had died as a result of wood alcohol poisoning. Whether the poisoning was accidental or homicidal was not clear. At the trial of the husband, the jury determined that the poisoning was accidental. "In all cases in which alcoholic poisoning is suspected, or which involve the discovery of alcoholic substances that may have been consumed, the crime laboratory should be requested to make analyses of samples of the liquids and also to determine blood alcohol content of victims."

COLLECTING SAMPLES FOR ALCOHOL ANALYSIS. There are a number of suggestions that may be useful in connection with the collection of samples of beverages containing alcohol. If mixed drinks are collected when there is ice still in the drink, the ice should be removed to prevent further dilution of the alcohol and any poisons that may be contained in it. The mixed liquid must be transferred to a chemically clean glass vial, which then is sealed tightly. The original glass container or other container should be processed for fingerprints. Obviously, it should be brought to the laboratory for further examination. Ideally, the container into which the unknown sample of liquor is transferred should be just large enough to hold the liquor, not oversized. If there is too much air space above the liquid sample, some of the alcohol will be lost by evaporation into that air space. Such evaporation could result in a higher value for a contained poison and could very well be the subject of cross-examination by the opposing attorney. "Blood alcohol examinations are usually conducted to determine the degree of intoxication. Blood samples must be carefully handled to prevent any loss of the volatile alcohol. Three to five cc of the blood are required."

BLOOD SAMPLES FOR ALCOHOL ANALYSIS. It is important that blood taken in order to ascertain the amount of blood alcohol should be drawn by qualified medical personnel. If at all possible, the investigator of the case should be present at the drawing.

Often, if the investigator is actually present, the doctor, nurse, or laboratory technician need not be called as a witness. The container in which the blood is put should have inscribed on it the name of the person who drew the sample. This information is critical if the investigator is not physically present when the sample was collected. The person taking the sample must be instructed not to use alcohol to sterilize the skin, nor must alcohol be used to sterilize the needles or other instruments used to make the collection. The investigator should instruct the medical personnel that the blood sample should be placed in a sealed, chemically clean test tube containing anticoagulant. The following cautions should be observed. Chemically clean containers should be used for all samples. The volume of air above the liquid sample must be minimal. The container holding the unknown sample must be sealed tightly. The container must be properly and completely marked.

METHODS. It is suggested that readers who wish to delve more deeply into how toxicologists carry out their studies and tests will find the book edited by Paget (1970) useful. Reid (1976) has reviewed methods for identifying drugs and trace materials in biological fluids. Choulis (1976) discusses the identification of drugs of abuse. Radioimmunassay has come into its own as a proven method for use by the forensic toxicologist (Castro and Malkus, 1977).

TIME. Poisons vary with respect to how quickly they act. Table 2-I shows the lethal times for various common poisons.

The Forensic Autopsy

The critical importance of a thorough and competent autopsy is nowhere better emphasized than in cases of poisoning and suspected poisoning.

The present widespread and seemingly unerasable attitudes of morticians and funeral directors with respect to autopsies and their role in human welfare conflict directly with the best professional practice to use in all death investigations; in poisoning cases their attitudes are in too many instances disastrous, for example, the federal report on the funeral industry (Severo, 1978).

Table 2-I
LETHAL TIME FOR VARIOUS COMMON POISONS*

Poison	Minimum Lethal Dose	LT_{50}
Cyanide	2 minutes	15 minutes
Strychnine	5 minutes	30 minutes
Organic phosphates	5 minutes	30 minutes
Formalin	10 minutes	35 minutes
Lysol	5 minutes	4 hours
Sulfuric acid	30 minutes	5 hours
Potassium dichromate	1 hour	5 hours
Nitric acid	2 hours	5 hours
Hydrochloric acid	10 minutes	9 hours
Arsenic	5 hours	11 hours
Methanol (wood alcohol)	4 hours	20 hours
Sodium hydroxide	1 hour	24 hours
Phosphorus	1 hour	24 hours
Mercury bichloride	1 hour	40 hours
Hypnotics		
Ethinamate	3 hours	15 hours
Bromovalerylurea	3 hours	27 hours
Barbiturate	3 hours	32 hours
Glutethimide	5 hours	42 hours

*Lethal time is the period between ingestion of poison and death. Minimum lethal dose is the smallest amount ever reported to have killed a human being. The LT_{50} is the time it takes for 50 percent of the persons ingesting a fatal dose of the poison to die (Watanabe, 1968).

The embalming procedure not only distorts the appearance of organs, tissues, wounds, and lesions, but it introduces under high pressures a mixture of poisonous chemicals into the corpse. These chemicals can obscure the results of analytical tests and frequently make such tests impossible. The "cleaning up" of the corpse inevitably washes away materials that may have important diagnostic value for the pathologist who does the autopsy (Wilber, 1974).

It might be appropriate to review briefly the reason for carrying out a forensic autopsy. First of all, the procedure should help to ascertain the cause and manner of death and is designed to throw some light on the time of death. In addition, the pathologist recovers, identifies, and preserves material of value as evidence in any legal action that may be justified on the basis of all the facts surrounding the case. Many facts surrounding the death may need to be tied together and interpreted; the forensic autopsy does just that. Of great importance is the production of a factual medical report, based on the autopsy findings, that can be used by all responsible officers in the criminal justice system, including defense lawyers. A proper forensic autopsy serves to protect the innocent by distinguishing natural deaths from unnatural deaths.

Lukash (Wilber, 1978) has outlined the procedures that are part of a competent medicolegal investigation of death:

1. Examination of the body before removal of clothing to note the condition of the clothing, to correlate defects and tears with obvious injuries, and to record artifacts.
2. Protection of clothing, body and hands against possible contamination prior to subsequent specific examination.
2. Recording of the general state of the body and clothing.
4. Observation of the extent of rigor mortis and lividity.
5. Recording of the temperature of the body and environment and any other data pertinent to subsequent determination of the time of death.
6. Notation of the date, time, and place of the autopsy procedure and the name of the examiner.
7. Notation of observers present.
8. Photographs used to identify the body and for reference in identifying specific injuries; also to demonstrate and to correlate external injuries with internal injuries.
9. Use of X-ray, which is important in locating bullets or other radiopaque objects for identification of the victim and for documentation of old fractures or anatomical deformities such as metallic foreign plates, nails, or screws.
10. Labeling all evidentiary items such as bullets or pellets for proper identification.
11. Preserving all tissue, fluids, and hair samples for further histological, bacteriological, histochemical, chemical, and toxicological examination.

Item 11 is of special importance in cases of poisoning. After the gross autopsy procedures have been completed, a battery of special laboratory tests must be performed on the biological materials taken as samples at the autopsy. These tests include microscopic tissue examination, chemical analyses, blood studies, serology, radiobiological tests, and in some instances bacteriological tests. These essential procedures are disrupted when the corpse from which the samples were taken has been embalmed.

Failure to take adequate samples at autopsy for later laboratory analysis may force an exhumation at some later date. Although modern technology has developed to a state where meaningful tests can be made on exhumed remains that are a decade old or more, such tests are a necessity forced on the forensic scientist by some past oversight by a pathologist, investigating officer, or other responsible official. The weight of such tests obviously is less than the weight of tests done before embalming or burial.

Law enforcement officers should have clearly in mind the fundamental need for a competent and thorough autopsy, including all appropriate laboratory tests, in all suspicious deaths that may involve poisoning. There is a classic example of a mass poisoner who carried out an unbelievable number of killings simply because each one was inadequately investigated and involved no autopsy.

Jolly Jane Toppan, a self-proclaimed nurse from Cambridge, Massachusetts, managed to murder at least thirty-one persons by poisoning while "nursing" them through illnesses or in old age. Her stepparents were her first victims. She was finally caught after wiping out a large part of the Davis family of Cataumet on Cape Cod. A suspicious grandfather who complained to an alert local physician exposed Jane. Her poison was a mixture of morphine and atropine, which left few external signs of poisoning to signal a physician asked to sign a death certificate. Apparently, none of the thirty-one deceased was subjected to an autopsy. The dead members of the Davis family were exhumed only after suspicions were aroused by the complaining grandfather.

REGISTRY OF HUMAN TOXICOLOGY. This registry is a useful reference facility for toxicologists who need to interpret analytical data for use in a court of law.

A recent study of a computer printout from the registry gives important information for the period of 1970 to 1975. In the United States, forty deaths due to ethanol were included in the registry files. The mean blood alcohol value for these deaths was 467 mg/100 ml of blood, with a range of 300 to 690 mg/100 ml and a standard deviation of ± 92 mg/100 ml. Deaths from carbon monoxide were the most frequently reported fatalities filed in the registry. The average value for all the fatal carbon monoxide cases was 65% saturation, with a range of 30 to 100% saturation and a standard deviation of 16% saturation.

The mean amount of ethanol, carbon monoxide, and barbiturates respectively in blood at death was consistent; the ranges were not wide.

The ranges for lethal amounts of morphine, propoxyphene, and amitryptiline respectively in blood were wide. For the latter drug (twenty-five deaths reported), the mean lethal blood content was 0.96 mg/100 ml; the range, 0.06 to 6.6 mg/100 ml.

Reference standards such as these are essential to a vigorous and effective program in forensic toxicology. Efforts should be made to insure that such an activity as the registry is kept up-to-date and functional.

Some Facts and Interpretations in Forensic Toxicology

At the present time, there are probably about 10,000 deaths each year as a result of poisoning. In 1968, for example, 3 percent of accidental deaths were due to poisons; 26 percent of the people who committed suicide used poisons. This 26 percent excludes the attempted suicides. Data from a wide variety of jurisdictions indicate that between fifteen and twenty cases of attempted suicide occur for every successful suicide. It then becomes obvious that a total of over 1 million nonfatal poisonings occur each year.

For suicidal use, the poisons of choice seem to be the derivatives of barbituric acid. Of the individuals who committed suicide by using drugs 75 percent used some sort of barbiturates.

In California in 1969, 54 percent of the suicides were carried out by the use of barbiturates, 17 percent by inhalation of the exhaust from automobiles, .7 percent by the use of salicylates, .4 percent by use of arsenic, and .5 percent by strychnine.

Accidental deaths showed a somewhat different percentage. In accidents, 20 percent of the fatalities resulted from barbiturates, and another 20 percent from the intake of opium compounds. Of accidental deaths, 2 percent occurred as a result of inhaling the exhaust from automobiles and about 1 percent from salicylates. The roles of arsenic and strychnine in accidental poisonings are not known from the data available.

Ethyl alcohol is not a first-line lethal chemical. It is, however, a widely used toxic chemical of grave concern to the toxicologist and to all law enforcement personnel. Repeated studies in various states across the United States have shown that at least 50 percent of the motor vehicle traffic deaths can be associated with elevated amounts of ethyl alcohol in the bodies of the victims.

A large but unknown percentage of the victims of homicide, suicide, and accidents have amounts of alcohol in their bodies that suggest intoxication. Because of the serious relationship between violent death and elevated alcohol levels in victims and in suspects, alcohol examination is probably the test most frequently carried out by the forensic toxicologist.

Role of the Forensic Toxicologist

The role of the forensic toxicologist in law enforcement matters is a severely demanding one. The forensic toxicologist is called upon to carry out sophisticated chemical analyses using modern equipment and techniques; but more than that, he is asked to perform these tests with speed, sensitivity, and a high degree of specificity. Because his results will be presented in court and will be subjected to vigorous cross-examination, the demands on him are indeed severe.

Despite the fact that the demands on the forensic toxicologist in modern day America are truly enormous, there is not an overall satisfactory program for educating forensic toxicologists. The fact that the American Academy of Forensic Sciences has an ongoing rigorous program of certification for forensic toxicologists suggests that the quality standards in that expert area are indeed commendable.

POLICY SUPPORT OF THE TOXICOLOGIST. All persons in the law enforcement system should realize that certain tissues are needed whenever a case of poisoning results. The investigating officers assigned to the case should be familiar with the needs of the toxicologist for biological material. The forensic pathologist certainly knows what is required, although the ordinary pathologist may not be familiar with the requirements. In such cases, the investigating officer assigned to the case should make specific requests of the pathologist to collect certain tissues under certain conditions. One of these conditions is that tissues taken from the body of a suspected poisoning victim should not be preserved by formaldehyde, alcohol, or any other chemical. These tissues should be put in a chemically clean glass jar and refrigerated. The toxicologist then can take it from there.

The toxicologist also needs a complete copy of the autopsy report. Many of the observations made at the autopsy table will be of crucial help to the toxicologist in arriving at the battery of tests he should perform to help in the investigation of a poisoning incident.

SIZE OF SAMPLE FOR ANALYSIS. An important point to remember in the collection of sample material for the forensic toxicologist is to *take enough*. When in doubt, take everything that is available. If not sure whether a piece of liver is needed or the whole liver, ask that the whole liver be taken. The toxicologist can always discard the excess if he does not need it. It is important to take adequate sizes of samples of all tissues from the body. In this way, one can circumvent the necessity for disinterring the body in case the chemical tests reveal the need for additional tissue.

If chronic metal poisoning may be the tentative cause of death, hair and fingernail specimens should be collected and put into separate containers. Fatty tissue is so easy to collect that it should be taken almost routinely. Pesticides, for example, accumulate in fat tissues, as do other chemicals. At autopsy, 50 gm of fat can be taken from underneath the skin, from around the kidneys, or from both without any great difficulty.

The toxicologist must keep in mind during this entire procedure that he is going to be faced with several questions concerning the poisoning situation. First of all, he must answer whether he found any poison. If the answer is affirmative, he then must answer specifically what poison was found. When these questions are answered, he then must come up with an answer to when the poison got into the victim's body and how the poison was found in the various tissues of the body and in the body as a whole. These questions all lead up to the important question of whether the amounts of the poisonous substances found are compatible with death being caused by their presence.

REPORT FORMS. There are various forms used by toxicologists to report the results of a toxicological examination. Ideally, most jurisdictions have a uniform report so that the investigating officers, the pathologists, district attorney, and others involved in a poisoning case can readily understand what the report means. Whenever the opportunity presents itself, law enforcement personnel should let the toxicologist know what information they need and in what form they need it. In this way, it may be possible for the toxicologist to design his formal report in such a way that it has the greatest value for the law enforcement process.

TESTIMONY. The toxicologist will necessarily be called as an expert witness to explain to the court the details of his examination and the opinions he formed as a result of these examinations. Law enforcement officers should understand that the toxicologist functions as an expert witness. He is *not* an advocate under any interpretation. His role is to uncover the facts of the case and to relate them to the court. Any conclusions and opinions he presents must be based on the facts that he has collected himself. He is not a partisan in the court case. He may be subpoenaed by the prosecution or by the defense. However, his testimony is for the court and must not be partial to either side in the trial.

It is important that an adequate pretrial conference occur between the expert and the lawyer who is trying the case. Law enforcement officers should themselves insure that such pretrial conference does in fact take place in any case in which they are involved. The investigating officer should not feel alarmed, insecure, nor hostile when the toxicologist, as an expert witness, permits the defense to interview him before a trial. It is desirable that the forensic toxicologist demonstrate complete impartiality with respect to the prosecution or defense. It is only with that firm attitude that he can function effectively in our court system. The defense and the prosecution both have a right to interview the expert witness before the actual testimony occurs. Remember that the forensic toxicologist, as an expert witness, is interested in truth as he has been able to uncover it as a result of his expert analyses.

REFERENCE SUPPORT. The forensic toxicologist has at his command a variety of resources that indicate that the future of that specialty will advance in a most positive way. The National Library of Medicine, for example, has a toxicology information program prepared to disseminate poisoning information through computerized retrieval of technical papers from the published literature. (Incidentally, there is a comparable program in Great Britian through the home office central research establishment.) These agencies use computer retrieval of analytical and other data of interest to toxicologists. There is also a registry of human toxicology sponsored by the American Academy of Forensic Sciences that is concerned with toxicological data, but especially that related to fatal cases.

There are real problems with respect to the retrieval and analysis of toxicological data. The absolute deluge of potentially dangerous new chemical agents requires highly sophisticated methods for storing data, retrieving it, and making it available to toxicologists generally.

INSTRUMENTATION. One of the remarkable developments in toxicology is the exquisite sophistication of instrumentation. Much of the outstanding advance in forensic toxicology can be traced directly to instrumentation. The procedure of combining various sophisticated instruments into a train, as it were, plus computerization of output indicate that there will be more rapid definitive analyses from forensic science laboratories in the future.

As a result of the significant advances made in clinical laboratory analyses through the process of automation, forensic science laboratories are beginning to explore the matter of automated analysis. From Great Britain have recently come reports of an automated procedure for the extraction, identification, and quantitative analysis of twenty samples for various drugs in an hour.

The automation of analytical procedures will bring some interesting problems into the courtroom. In an automated procedure such as one can do for blood sugar and other analyses of body fluids, who actually did the analysis? How does a lawyer cross-examine an automation? Will the courts permit data obtained almost completely by automation to be introduced into evidence? If such data are admitted, what will be the restrictions, who will testify, and how can the cross-examination be carried out? These and other questions will have to be solved by repeated court decisions; eventually, some form of acceptance will become widespread.

The Problem of So-Called Subclinical Poisoning Effects

The term *subclinical* is one that deserves to be erased from the vocabulary of toxicologists. Its meaning is vague. The mischief that its use causes is unacceptable. In connection with lead toxicity, a recent study defines subclinical poisoning by lead as follows: "Recently the concept of subclinical lead poisoning has been elaborated and this may be defined as the production of morbidity or mortality without the appearance of the classical signs or symptoms of clinical lead poisoning" (Waldron and Stofen, 1974) .

This definition illustrates the confusion generated by the use of the term subclinical. It is not readily apparent how death cannot be recognized as a definite illness. It is also not clear how death can be an early stage of an illness. If this term is used in litigation, it is the author's opinion that it can be demolished by appropriate questioning in an attempt to clarify the phrase.

If one takes the definition for lead poisoning given by Waldron and Stofen (1974) and compares it with their definition for subclinical poisoning, the confusion becomes obvious. They define lead poisoning as follows: "Lead poisoning may be metabolic or clinical. Metabolic poisoning may be said to be present when it is possible to detect alterations in metabolism which are the result of lead absorption. Clinical lead poisoning is diagnosed when the absorbed lead produces signs or symptoms which are evident to the patient or his doctor. Metabolic poisoning may exist without clinical poisoning but not the converse." Apparently from this definition combined with the definition of subclinical lead poisoning, the situation of being "not long for this world" is not a sign or symptom of anything. In addition, death is apparently not a sign of anything that would point to a clinical disease.

In a most informed discussion of the problem of subclinical effects of chemicals, Palmes (1976) has pointed out a number of facts and considerations that are important in any evaluation of poisoning, from pesticides, for example. The so-called subclinical effects are important because they indicate exposure to some specific chemical. These effects do not imply that a process of disease has been initiated. Moreover, there is no implication that the exposure will inevitably bring about the most grave effect the agent can produce in man, in animals, or in the test tube.

An indication that there has been exposure to a small but measurable amount of a chemical in no way forces the conclusion that the most serious consequences the chemical in question can produce will necessarily follow. As Palmes points out, "Exposure is not equivalent to poisoning." Death is obviously the gravest effect that can result from exposure to some chemical. As a general rule, there is some dose or concentration of virtually any material that kills some percentage of animals that have been exposed to the agent in question. In addition, there is a clear probability that some dose lower than the first kills a smaller percentage of animals that are exposed to the agent.

If we extrapolate this to man, some percentage of human beings will be killed by exposure to that chemical. Palmes (1976) points out the strange anomaly: "This risk of death is usually acceptable while that of carcinogenesis or other chronic and ultimately fatal disease is not." Specifically, "If exposure is measurable at any level and if carcinogenesis is a toxic property of the agent, the agent is likely to be banned. If the agent only produces mortality, it might still be acceptable at what are judged to be sublethal levels" (Palmes, 1976) .

Commonly Employed Toxicology Analytic Techniques*

Gas liquid chromatography (GLC) is an analytic technique by which drugs may be separated by partitioned chromatography at a high temperature. The tentative identification of drugs may be made by comparing unknowns with the chromatographic behavior of pure drug standards.

Thin layer chromatography (TLC) is an analytic technique by which drugs may be separated by adsorption chromatography on 0.5 mm thin sheets of adsorbent. Extracted drugs are applied to the thin sheets along with drug standards, and these drug mixtures are separated with organic solution as they are moved along the thin sheet. Tentative identification is made by comparison with standards, as well as observing the unique color of the drug that develops after spraying the separated drugs with specific color reagents.

Ultraviolet spectroscopy (UV) is an absorption technique that allows identification of purified drugs in solution. Each drug molecule absorbs ultraviolet light in a unique fashion; by comparing the pattern of absorption with a drug standard, the UV technique can be used to confirm the presence and quantity of drug in the sample.

A co-oximeter is a spectrophotometric instrument designed to specifically measure absorption of visible light by the hemoglobin molecule. The degree of light absorption by the molecule changes as the hemoglobin combines with increasing amounts of carbon monoxide. By monitoring this change in light absorption, the instrument gives a direct reading of the percent saturation of hemoglobin by carbon monoxide.

---

*Courtesy of James T. Weston, M.D., Editor, *Newsletter,* Office of the Medical Investigator, State of New Mexico, Albuquerque, New Mexico.

Chapter 3

SUICIDE

General Comments

SUICIDE IS A PHENOMENON that reaches into all economic levels, races, ages, nationalities, and sexes (Wilber, 1974). Each year there are more reported suicides and suicide attempts than the previous year. In the neighborhood of 25,000 suicides are recorded in the United States each year. "The number of suicides in the United States are [*sic*] more than the total deaths caused by scarlet fever, diphtheria, whooping cough, malaria, typhoid fever, measles, typhus, meningoccal infections, infantile paralysis, rheumatic fever, and bronchitis" (Faivre, 1978).

Some Guidance

A person who threatens suicide or debates it as an option in his life must be taken seriously. Of those who commit suicide, 80 percent have given a warning signal of their proposed act. Many suicides, but not all, can be prevented. Of recorded suicides, 80 percent are carried out by persons who have made at least one previous attempt. A repeated attempt usually takes place about ninety days after the subject seems to have recovered from an attempt and appears adjusted.

Suicide is not a genetic disease. It is not inherited like brown eyes, for example. However, some families seem to have more suicides in them than others. Home conditions may be a partial explanation.

The conclusion that everyone who commits suicide is insane (whatever "insane" really means) cannot be supported by available facts. Many who commit suicide are depressed and can see "no light at the end of the tunnel." Others are in a biological state such that they see reality and respond to it differently than do most people. When they are in such a state, self-destruction is to them the logical, and indeed may seem to be the only correct, option for them to take.

Most suicides happen late in the afternoon or early in the evening. About 85 percent of all suicides in the United States are *not* accompanied by a suicide note.

RELIGION. Judaism considers suicide to be unacceptable as a breaking of the decalogue. Christianity, certainly after the time of St. Augustine, viewed suicide as a sin for the person involved. Catholics today look upon suicide as sinful for the victim and for anyone who cooperates in the act. As a practical matter, Catholics presume that anyone who does away with himself was at the time of the act not in complete mental control of the situation. Hence, Catholic suicides are no longer denied a Christian burial. Many other Christian groups today leave the question of suicide an open one.

SEX. Three times as many women attempt suicide as do men. Completed suicides are comprised of 70 percent men and 30 percent women. Men usually use the more potent forms of self-killing: firearms, hanging, defenestration, and one-car automobile crashes. Women in general avoid methods of suicide that will disfigure them (Wilber, 1974).

SUICIDE-PRONE. Two classes of individuals are among those who are especially susceptible to committing suicide:

1. Alcoholics who have exhibited uncontrolled ethanol intake for a long time
2. Chronic abusers of drugs

SEDATIVE AND HYPNOTIC DRUGS. Sedative and hypnotic drugs are widely used with and without prescription. They are readily obtained by most adults who want them. Presumably their action, even to fatality, is painless. For these reasons, this group of drugs provides favorite tools in many countries for suicide. In the United States, barbiturates and tranquilizers are usually the instruments of choice for suicide, especially by women.

Treatment of these drug suicide attempts requires skilled medical attention provided as rapidly as possible. The suicide victims in these cases are usually unconscious or semiconscious when the rescue services or the police are called. Treatment involves the following:

1. Removal of drug from the body
2. Counteracting the depressing action of these drugs on vital centers in the body (control centers in the brain for respiration and circulation of blood)
3. Prevention of coma that lasts for a long time

In modern, well-equipped hospitals, it is not necessary to wash out from the stomach all unabsorbed remains of swallowed drugs. Artificial kidney machines used in conjunction with appropriate medication can increase the excretion of harmful drug excesses from the body by a factor of four.

Poisons and Suicide

STATISTICS ON SUICIDE.   Much of the statistical information about violent, unattended, and suspicious deaths is less than satisfactory. The statistics on suicide share this fault. Suicides are probably underreported as a mode of death. The determination of suicide in cases of poisonings is especially difficult because accidental exposures are not infrequent; the process of separating accidental from suicidal poisonings is tedious and not always effective.

Psychotropic drugs (those that act on the brain so as to modify consciousness) are instruments that are used in a number of suicides (McGuire et al., 1976). In a study of four major cities in the United States (Washington, Miami, Dallas, and San Francisco), the mean age of individuals who used these agents for suicide was 38 to 46; the mean age for nonsuicidal deaths from psychotropic drugs was 27 to 35 years. Of the totals, 68 to 90 percent were white; 0 to 29 percent were black. But, there is still a haziness about the data (Table 3-I) .

What drugs are used in suicides? In general, 51 percent of the deaths that are suicidal involve barbiturates as the agent. The value varies from a high of 75 percent in San Francisco to a low of 30 percent in Dallas. In general, narcotics are *not* used suicidally.

Table 3-I
PSYCHOTROPIC DRUG DEATHS

Definitely suicide	36 percent
Probable suicide	7 percent
Possible suicide	3 percent
Suspicious	7 percent
Not suicide	44 percent
Unknown	3 percent

Nonsuicidal drug deaths in Washington, D.C. show that 92 percent of them are from narcotics, whereas in Miami only 23 percent of these deaths are caused by narcotics. Heroin or morphine make up 23 percent of all nonsuicidal narcotic deaths; in 25 to 40 percent of these cases, alcohol is abused simultaneously.

Additional information is given about the characteristics of psychotropic drug deaths in Tables 3-II and 3-III.

Table 3-II
SEXUAL DIFFERENCES IN FREQUENCY OF PSYCHOTIC DRUG DEATHS*

City	Suicidal		Nonsuicidal	
	Males	Females	Males	Females
Washington	40	60	86	14
Miami	45	55	63	37
Dallas	53	47	68	32
San Francisco	48	52	71	29
Overall	46	54	75	25

*Values are in percentages.

Table 3-III
SUICIDE AND OCCUPATION*

Occupational Level	Suicidal	Nonsuicidal
Professional	21	4
Semiprofessional	18	7
Skilled	20	14
Semiskilled	21	25
Unskilled	20	50

*The values are the same for all cities shown in Table 3-II.

Confirmed by toxicologic analysis of blood and urine, 385 suicide attempts by drug ingestion were investigated over a thirteen-month period. There were 275 cases of drug overdoses, including 2 deaths. Drugs ingested in order of frequency included (1) barbiturates, (2) nonprescriptive drugs, (3) alcohol, (4) glutethimide, (5) miscellaneous prescription drugs, and (6) poisons. Mixed drug overdoses (usually two compounds) resulted in 3 deaths out of 110 patients. Alcohol was involved in two-thirds of the mixed drug cases, including the 3 fatal cases. It is suggested that gluthethimide, present in 9 percent of the attempts including all 5 deaths, never be prescribed in an amount large enough to be fatal in one dose (Holland et al., 1975).

PESTICIDE SUICIDES. In south Florida, suicides made up 51 to 72 percent of fatalities from all poisons for every year from 1956 to 1967 inclusive. During this twelve-year span, 121 deaths were caused by pesticides, 57 percent of these deaths were suicidal, and 10 percent were murders (Reich et al., 1968).

The epidemiology of the suicides was unique:

> Average age at suicide, 46 years
> Percentage of blacks, 20 percent
> Man-to-woman ratio, about 1:1
> Use of organic phosphates, 39 percent

In all probability, the incidence of suicides in this study is under-reported, as is true for most suicide data.

In the United States, it is unusual for suicide or murder to be carried out using the newer pesticides as poisons. In foreign countries, a different situation obtains. During 1954, at least 75 suicides and murders were carried out by the use of parathion in Germany. In Finland between 1955 and 1957, 219 suicides by parathion poisoning were recorded. In Japan in the years 1953 and 1954, parathion caused hundreds of deaths (a total of 1500 cases of poisonings by parathion were recorded). Suicides by use of parathion accounted for 500 deaths each year in Japan from 1955 through 1960.

DEATHS IN GARAGES. Deaths in garages are frequently suicidal in nature. However, they are not always straightforward and thus pose extra investigative work for the police officers involved. Not only is it important to pinpoint the cause and manner of death in order to exclude homicide as a possibility, but it is also critical that adequate information be on record in the event that the case has insurance, liability, civil suit, inheritance, or other ramifications. Could next of kin sue the investigating officers for abridgment of civil rights or for neglect of equal protection under the law in the event the investigation is not "adequate"? For good reasons, then, Weston (1976) opines that "deaths in garages cause more problems than any other category we see."

The following example illustrates the complexity of a "simple" death in a garage. According to the medical investigator's report, a fifty-five-year-old executive killed himself by inhalation of fumes from an auto exhaust. He was found by his wife when she returned home unexpectedly. Although she rushed into the garage and attempted to retrieve her warm, limp husband from the garage, he was dead on arrival at the hospital emergency room. The wife described to the medical examiner a despondent male who was recovering from major surgery and had a problem of alcoholism.

The blood carbon monoxide level was only 5% to 10%, a fact that caused some puzzlement until an autopsy was finished, including a more thorough toxicological report. The latter showed the following: carbon monoxide, 35% saturation; alcohol, 0.17 gm/100 ml of blood; pentobarbital, 0.3 mg/100 ml of blood.

The husband had a group accidental death insurance policy worth $150,000 among his effects. Apparently the wife had not known about the policy, but the insurance company did and was not about to pay off unless accidental death could be clearly proven.

According to the wife, her husband had been working in the garage, as was not unusual. In cold weather, he ran the car engine to keep warm inside the unheated garage. She was unable to remember exactly where her husband was and where the car was when she found the victim. Ambulance attendants were unsure just where the various work tools were located when they arrived; the wife did not agree with their vague impression. She could not recall pulling her husband out of the garage. Moreover, there apparently had been a note of some sort scribbled by the deceased on a torn anniversary card and found in the bedroom by the wife. She claimed that the scrap had presumably been thrown out with trash. Here is a case with insurance ramifications and some critical details that are hazy enough to cause generalized discontent with what could finally be done about the case.

The deceased had been afflicted with a bleeding stomach ulcer; he had had surgery and was recovering from it. Obviously he was anemic. The technician who did the first carbon monoxide test noticed that the blood sample was mostly plasma, with comparatively few red cells; no correction was made for the actual amount of hemoglobin in the sample. After autopsy, the blood sample obtained was closer to normal hemoglobin concentration; a hemoglobin correction factor was also used. The resulting 35% saturation value was probably fairly close to the correct value. This episode indicates the necessity of having *all* analytical data listed in a toxicology report. Specifically, in this case, the measured hemoglobin in the blood sample should have been recorded and reported, as should have been the hemoglobin correction factor used. A blood sample that has little red coloring matter in it is useless for carbon monoxide measurements. Whenever a low carbon monoxide value is found in a test when surrounding circumstances suggest carbon monoxide poisoning, the measured hemoglobin in the sample must be reported and recorded. The minimal carbon monoxide level to cause death is about 40 to 50%.

Weston summarizes the poisoning situation for small closed spaces: "Auto exhaust fumes may produce 3 lbs. of carbon monoxide for every gallon of gas burned. Since CO has a 240-260 times greater affinity for Hb than oxygen, even a low carbon monoxide concentration may prove rapidly fatal. This is particularly true with a rapid respiratory rate, significant coronary disease or, as in this case, alcohol and drug sedation. A fatal CO level accumlates in a closed, single-car garage with a running auto in about 5-10 minutes."

Garage deaths are serious business. The ramifications are at times astonishing. Therefore, it seems important that an investigating officer and a deputy medical examiner or deputy coroner actually visit the scene to insure that adequate documentation (sketches and photographs) is obtained about position of any tools, work space size and layout, broken windows, and condition of garage doors and locks. Originals of all so-called suicide notes must be kept in the case file. The family should be given copies as they wish, but the original must never be released. It is part of the permanent investigative record. Some day one of these original suicide notes will prove to be a pearl beyond price. Ideally, all statements that are originally made by next of kin or witnesses should be recorded accurately; if at all possible, magnetic tape recordings should be made of these initial statements. Tape recorders that use standard cassettes and are rugged enough for police use can be purchased for about $40 each. Their quality of reproduction is excellent. Microcassette tape recorders are costly for the most part (anywhere from $300 to $700 per unit), although a few inexpensive ones are available and perform well with care. Tape recorders are an important part of an investigator's armamentarium. Tape recordings can prove to be a most impressive form of evidence.

VARIATION OF GARAGE DEATHS. A recent case comes to mind of a public servant in his fifties who was found dead in his living room, which was located over a built-in garage. He had a flushed facial appearance. Examination of the garage showed that the car engine had been running; ignition key was on; gasoline tank was empty; door from garage to kitchen was open. The man's blood CO was about 20%, but further blood toxicological tests showed that he was legally drunk and his blood contained well over the therapeutic levels of Librium® and Valium®. Careful questioning of his widow and daughter established without doubt that the death was self-engineered.

A similar case comes to mind of a couple in their seventies who went to bed in the usual fashion but left the car running in the garage (attached to the kitchen side of the house) with the door between garage and kitchen left open; all other doors to the outside were closed and locked. Carbon monoxide from the fumes emanating from the garage entered the kitchen, got into the heating system cold air return, and then was distributed throughout the house, including the bedroom where the man and wife were sleeping. Careful examination of all aspects of the case combined with the results of careful autopsies on both victims led to the conclusion that this was a case of a suicide pact successfully carried out.

ALCOHOL AND SUICIDE. The suicidal bent of alcoholic persons is a serious risk to driving safety in the United States as well as in other countries (Bartholomew, 1967).

Suicide is more frequent among alcoholics than it is in the general population (Goodwin, 1973). Strangely enough, alcoholism is more common among those who attempt suicide (but fail) than it is among those who commit suicide. There is evidence that alcoholic females have higher rates of suicide and attempted suicide than do alcoholic men (Kinsey, 1966; Schuckit, 1972).

Menninger (1938) postulated that alcoholism is a form of self-destruction; it is slow suicide. Studies since that time tend to support this postulate (Rushing, 1969).

Physicians, compared to the general population, have a high rate of suicide (Wilber, 1974). Among them 40 percent of the suicides are associated with alcoholism (National Clearinghouse for Alcohol Information, 1974).

The available literature strongly supports the contention that alcoholism as a cause of suicide is not unique to any nation, race, class of society, or sex, but is a common relationship in *Homosapiens* (National Clearinghouse for Alcohol Information, 1974).

Table 3-IV, listing common chemicals and their effective levels, may be useful.

Table 3-IV
BLOOD LEVEL

Chemical	Use	Therapeutic	Lethal
Amobarbital (Amytal®)	Sedative-hypnotic	2 mg %	6 mg %
Aspirin	Pain relief	30 mg %	More than 70 mg %
Butisol®	Hypnotic	3 mg %	Over 5 mg %
Librium®	Tranquilizer	0.25 mg %	*MLD @ 2 grams
Valium®	Tranquilizer	0.03 mg %	MLD @ 1 gram
Doriden®	Sedative	2 mg %	MLD @ 10 grams
Miltown®	Tranquilizer	@ 1 mg %	@ 8 or more mg %
Morphine	Pain killer	—	0.5 mg %
Nembutal®	Sedative	1.5 mg %	4 mg %
Luminal®	Sedative	3-4 mg %	20 mg %
Seconal®	Sedative	1 mg %	3-5 mg %
Placidyl®	Sedative	1 mg %	6 mg %

*Minimum lethal dose.

Chapter 4

DRUGS OF ABUSE

IN DISCUSSING DRUG ABUSE, the term *addiction* is used. Addiction may be physical or it may be psychological. The general term addiction refers to a condition in which there is a periodic or long-term requirement for a repeated dose of a specific chemical. The individual who is addicted experiences an overwhelming desire or drive to continue taking a specific chemical; the drive is so strong that the goal of obtaining it makes acceptable virtually any means to get the drug. There is a tendency in the addicted individual to increase the dose; in other words, the drug in question builds up a tolerance in the addict. There may be, in the addicted individual, a psychological or a physiological need for the effects the drug exerts on the individual. Finally, the end result of such chemical abuse usually is harmful to the individual and to society.*

Physical addiction depends upon a physiological demand for a drug or other chemical brought about by frequent and repetitive use of that particular drug. When the drug in question is not available, a peculiar type of response known as *physical abstinence syndrome* occurs. This syndrome is composed of a number of withdrawal symptoms that include nausea and vomiting, sweating,

---

*There is a logical difficulty with the use of this widely accepted definition of addiction. It involves the use of the term *abuse* as well as the concept of *harm* to oneself or to society. These ideas are ethical in nature and not medical nor scientific. Virtually *all* definitions of addiction share this clear aspect of being moral or ethical statements, not declarations of scientific fact. Regrettable efforts are made to buttress these definitions by immoderate and falsifying attempts to overplay the actual physical harm caused to persons and communities by the use of so-called illicit drugs. Forensic scientists and law enforcement personnel must resist these falsifying endeavors.

general pain in the abdominal area with upset of the digestive tract, cramps and pains in the muscles, headaches, muscle tremors, general upset of the metabolism of the body, convulsions, and even death.

Psychological addiction is a conscious or mind-centered requirement for some chemical or drug. The need is not physical but may indeed become an extremely potent compulsion. Withdrawal symptoms are brought about in the victim when the chemical or drug is not available. These symptoms are included under the general title of *psychological abstinence syndrome*. This syndrome includes the following symptoms: generalized uneasiness, anxiety, panic, aggressive behavior that may even be criminal, delusions and hallucinations, psychosis, depression, and at times, suicide.

What chemicals cause psychological and physiological addiction? It has been demonstrated by actual experiments and clinical observations that the following kinds of drugs and chemicals can and do cause *physiological* addiction in man: narcotics, barbiturates, some tranquilizers, some amphetamines, alcohol, and tobacco. It has been maintained that ether, petroleum products, and some kinds of glue, because they are volatile agents and can be inhaled, do cause physiological addiction. The evidence for this is less than completely satisfactory. Drugs known to cause *psychological* addiction include: narcotics, barbiturates, some tranquilizers, amphetamines, hallucinogens, alcohol, marijuana, and tobacco. Ether, petroleum products, and glue are also said to cause psychological addiction at times. Again, the evidence in favor of these volatile agents causing psychological addiction is not overwhelmingly persuasive.

These comments are based on biomedical considerations. When one tries to compare the biomedical definitions of terms with the legal definitions, there are differences, and indeed, contradictions, that are hard to resolve. The toxicologist, of course, is concerned with the biomedical definitions of these various toxicological terms, but he works in an environment, especially when he is testifying, that uses the legal definitions. Consequently, he must make himself into an expert translator of medical definitions in toxicology and the legal definitions for the same terms. He has to be able to switch back and forth between the legal and the medical definitions quickly, smoothly, and competently.

An example of this problem can be given when one thinks of a central nervous system depressant. Medically, a central nervous system depressant is any agent that depresses the functions of the central nervous system. From a legal point of view, a central nervous system depressant is a drug that may produce any of the following: a calming effect or relief from emotional tension or anxiety; drowsiness, sedation, sleep, stupor, coma, or general anesthesia; increase in the threshold for pain; mood depression or apathy; and disorientation, confusion, or loss of mental acuity. Here we see that the legal definition in a sense throws every possible response into the pot, as it were, in order to produce a mechanism that will catch crooks.* The various elements of this mechanism may not be medically sound.

A Nontoxicological Note

The legal classification of drugs of abuse, especially the breakdown of narcotics, has caused much mischief. It is important to realize that the legal classification of drugs does not bear a precise relationship to the scientific classification of drugs. For example, cocaine in the United States is classified as a narcotic. Scientifically, cocaine is a stimulant and a local anesthetic. It is in no way a narcotic drug. On the other hand, all nations in the world classify cannabis (marijuana) and the chemical derivatives of

---

*So-called tough drug control laws have been consistently shown to fail in furthering the state objectives of such legislation. A recent in-depth study of the New York State anti–drug-abuse law made by the Joint Committee on New York Drug Law Evaluation (1977 1978A, 1978B) demonstrates that the goals of the law to control illegal drug use have not been achieved. Heroin abuse continued at the same high rate in New York City three years after the "Rockefeller Drug Law" was implemented as it was before the law was enacted. New York's pattern of drug-related crimes after the law was essentially the same as in nearby states having no such "tough" laws. The stiff penalties (monstrous, according to some legal experts) showed no sustained deterrent effects. The enormous costs forced on the state by the drug laws yielded no commensurate benefits. It should be clear that savage anti–drug-abuse laws savagely enforced degrade society but do nothing to cure the "abuse" of chemical substances.

marijuana as narcotic drugs. As far as can be ascertained at this time, there is no exception made in any country of the world with respect to the legal classification of cannabis as a narcotic. Scientifically, cannabis is listed as a mild depressant, but certainly not as a narcotic.

Toxicologists who are asked to testify on matters of drug abuse and to advise the court on scientific matters of drugs and pharmacology should be alert to the fact that the legal aspects of drug classification can be confusing when translating such classification into the scientific classification of the same drugs. It is important that this disparity be kept clearly in mind so that confusion between the expert toxicologist and the court can be kept to a minimum.

Classification of Drugs

The drugs that are prescription items, for the most part, and are abused so that problems of poisoning arise may be classified as follows:

I. Hypnotics
   A. Amobarbital
   B. Barbital
   C. Butabarbital
   D. Chloral hydrate
   E. Ethchlorvynol
   F. Flurazepam
   G. Glutethimide
   H. Meprobamate
   I. Methyprylon
   J. Pentobarbital
   K. Phenobarbital
   L. Secobarbital

II. Analgesics
   A. Meperidine
   B. Pentazocine
   C. Propoxyphene

     D. Salicylate

III. Psychotherapeutics
     A. Amitryptyline
     B. Chlorpromazine
     C. Chlordiazephoxide
     D. Diazepam
     E. Imipramine
     F. Promazine

IV. Anticonvulsants
     A. Diphenylhydantoin
     B. Primidone

V. Aliphatic alcohols
     A. Ethanol
     B. Isopropanol
     C. Methanol

Some General Facts on Drug Abuse in the United States

Approximately 43 million persons have smoked marijuana at least once to try it out. More than 16 million Americans are regular users of the weed. Nearly one-tenth of high school seniors smoke marijuana daily. A warning should be taken from the statistic that about 15 percent of automobile accidents in the United States today are related directly to intoxication with marijuana.

Cocaine, a stimulant, has been tried at least once by about 10 million Americans. Heroin addicts number almost 400,000 in the United States (compared with 9 million alcohol addicts); their number is decreasing.

Cocaine is not addicting, but many users become so attached to the results of its use that they center their lives on it in an unwholesome and ultimately self-destructive manner.

Use of marijuana poses a bevy of risks to individual health and to the welfare of society; among these risks are unhealthy self-centeredness, loss of social sense, decrease in sexual interest and performance, modification of hormone levels in the body and of the immunity mechanism, damage to the lungs, and prolonged half-life of tetrahydrocannabinol in the body. Laboratory data have demonstrated that marijuana will more probably cause tumors resembling cancer than will cigarette smoke. If marijuana were a pesticide (such as DDT) or a food additive (such as saccharin), the laboratory evidence available on it would force it to be banned by several federal agencies.

Phencyclidine (PCP) apparently has been used at least once by 14 percent of young people eighteen to twenty-five years of age. The use of this potent hallucinogen seems to be increasing; there is reported to be a 48 percent increase in PCP abuse from 1976 to 1977 in the eighteen– to twenty-five-year age-group. According to a claim made by the National Institute of Drug Abuse, more than 7 million Americans have used PCP at least once. PCP is also called *hog* or *angel dust*. It is frequently used with other drugs. A favorite method is to saturate marijuana with it and then smoke the mixture.

Reality of the Problem

The problem of evaluating the toxicology of the so-called drugs of abuse is compounded and confused by the nonsense, too often preached as absolute truth, that surrounds discussion of the drugs of abuse and of the legislation relating to them.

The crimes of drug abuse fall under the category of *malum prohibitum,* that is, actions that are criminal simply because of a statute. Drug abuse is not *malum in se,* that is, actions that are inherently unlawful such as murder, rape, or stealing.

Statutes create most of the crimes that fall under the category of drug abuse. *Malum prohibitum* crimes must be clearly outlined in painful detail because they are crimes "manufactured" by law. They must also be interpreted narrowly in the stated restrictions. Judicial ineptitude and legislative overkill have combined to confuse the complex of drug abuse laws *(malum prohibitum)* in a most disgraceful and unedifying manner.

The too common corrosion of integrity of law enforcement personnel, administrators, and judges who wade deeply or often in the swamp of drug law enforcement should stimulate critical analyses of just what we are after in our numerous drug abuse control endeavors.*

Alcohol

The drug that is most flagrantly abused by our society, and a drug that is also in and of itself insidiously poisonous, is ethyl alcohol (ethanol, grain alcohol, distilled spirits). Socially as well as legally, the abuse of alcohol is respectable; the alcohol addict (the alcoholic) is protected by a galaxy of laws and a growing throng of social workers. A peculiar social response to alcohol addiction prevails in the face of awful facts: the drug *alcohol* is the triggering agent for 50 to 65 percent of fatal automobile accidents every year; half of all arrests in the majority of United States cities are related to abuse of alcohol by the person arrested; 10 percent of the persons admitted to mental hospitals are alcohol abusers. "The alcoholic is a difficult person to handle; he is noisy, often pugnacious, frequently homicidal, in all ways a social menace" (Lee, 1972). In most jurisdictions his addiction is legally a disease, but treatment is not legally mandatory.

Morphine

The morphine or heroin addict is just the opposite; suppressed, pleasant, nonbelligerent, quiet, and afflicted with the "nods." If given a regular dose of opium derivative without fear or penalty, these opiate addicts can carry on normal activities for decades with *no* physical or mental deterioration.

Morphine and its various derivatives and synthetic substitutes are potently addicting; victims of the addiction must have a regular intake. Experience over decades, amply documented in voluminous medical records, has demonstrated that for all practical purposes, morphine addicts (including persons addicted to any opium derivative or substitute) are not curable. They have a real chronic sickness demonstrable chemically and physiologically. The

---

*Physicians lead in diversion of drugs. Since initiation by the federal government, Diversion Investigative Units (DIUs) have made over 1300 arrests involving medical and paramedical persons. Physicians (MDs) lead the list in arrests for diverting drugs to illicit traffic (*The Toxicology Newsletter,* 1977).

only therapy of proven value is maintenance doses of the addicting chemical. Legally, these sick patients must be cured or be branded as criminals.

Identification

Treatment of drug overdose cases includes rapid identification of the drug that is causing the toxic reactions. At least one manufacturer of drugs provides an identification code for its products. Unknown drugs or formulations from the company, even the unlabeled, can be rapidly identified by reference to the code pamphlet.†

Armed Forces

The fact that the problems of drug abuse are not merely academic is illustrated by the contention that the use of hard drugs is escalating, as of early 1978, among American servicemen at an alarming rate (Duncan, 1978).‡ It has been proposed that random urine tests of servicemen be reinstituted in an attempt to curb the increase. In 1976, Congress barred such tests as invasion of privacy. Some of the facts used to support the contention of increasing drug abuse among the United States military are summarized below.

Over 8 percent of soldiers in the Berlin Brigade (3500 men) admitted that they used heroin; 4 heroin overdose deaths occurred to Brigade personnel in 1977. There are 225,000 soldiers stationed in West Germany. Rumor has it that some of the United States units in that population have a heroin usage rate of up to 40 percent, although the validity of the estimate is of the lowest order.

On a Navy aircraft carrier, urine tests were done on sailors (samples were not identified as to specific source); 20 percent of

---

†Identi-Code® Index (formula identification code, Lilly), Eli Lilly Company, Indianapolis, Indiana 46206. Copies are available, at no cost, for retention in communication centers, investigative offices, laboratories, or hospital emergency rooms.
‡The civilian staff of the President of the United States seems to be involved in drug abuse deeply enough to move the President to order this staff to obey the laws of the land with respect to illegal use of drugs (Herron and Habermann, 1978)

the sailors tested were using heroin or some other opium derivative. It is not clear how many were using prescribed cough medicine containing codeine.

A random sample was taken of United States military personnel around the world; they were given a questionnaire covering a
number of topics. Of the 2350 individuals in the sample, nearly
one-third held that drug use in their particular units was at such
a high level that the units could not perform optimally in combat.
In the same survey, three-quarters of the officers responding expressed the belief that 50 percent of the low-ranking permanently
enlisted individuals used marijuana weekly; a smaller percentage
was said to use heroin now and then.

Random Urine Tests

The random urine test program is ineffective in meeting the
problem of drug abuse in the military.* Its value in curbing the
abuse of drugs is virtually zero; its capacity for alienating troops
and destroying morale is extremely high. It has such an air of
totalitarianism about it that it is not appropriate for an American
defense force kept in existence to protect "democracy" around the
world. Properly, the Department of Defense refused to start the
program again. The Department opts rather for a more useful
plan of giving officers the authority to order appropriate medical
tests for individual servicemen who seem to have problems related
to drug abuse.

This attitude on the part of the Department of Defense officials†
is refreshing because it puts the drug abuse problem where it be-
longs: in the hands of the medical profession. Our national
civilian experience over the decades has demonstrated beyond
challenge that handling the drug abuse situation as a police matter

---

*By the use of a host of standard clinical chemical tests subjected to appropriate
statistical treatment, it is said to be possible to distinguish a population of drug
abusers from a control population of nonabusers (the respective laboratory "profiles" vary). The error for the control group is 4 percent; for the abusers, 14
percent (Mayron et al., 1974).

†It is safe to say that drug abuse in the military as well as alcoholism and other
"anomalies" of behavior reflect the situation in the society from which the service
personnel are drawn. Service people are just more conspicuous.

is ineffective and so counterproductive that we have, by using the "law enforcement" approach, magnified the problem in the United States to a monstrous level (Weinraub, 1978).

A Survey of the More Commonly Abused Groups of Drugs
Marijuana

Marijuana, in its various forms, is second to alcohol as probably the most abused drug in the United States. The use of marijuana on a regular basis or occasionally is so widespread in every geographical area, and in virtually every age-group, that enforcement of laws against the abuse of this drug cannot be carried out in any meaningful way.

The reactions of individuals to marijuana originate from the chemical effect that the active agents in the smoke from the marijuana plant exert on the body, plus subjective effects that occur as a result of the setting or surroundings in which the individual is carrying out ritual smoking; the expectations of the individual using marijuana subjectively bring on certain reactions. Past experience, obviously, will have some meaning on what the subject thinks is happening to him. The potency of the various marijuana preparations available in the United States varies widely. Consequently, the effects an individual gets from smoking marijuana will vary in an unpredictable way.

It is important for law enforcement officers to understand clearly that no physical dependence has ever been demonstrated for marijuana, even when it is used excessively. Whether tolerance develops or not is not clear. In isolated instances, there seems to be a suggestion that a tolerance to the drug may, in fact, occur. Psychological dependence seems to occur in a number of individuals. In other words, marijuana can become a crutch. However, this kind of dependence is not unique to marijuana, but is found among individuals who become dependent on coffee, tea, and tobacco smoke. When an individual is withdrawn from marijuana use, there is no indication of the abstinence syndrome or the withdrawal effects. There seems to be no evidence of organic damage to the human body as a result of using marijuana other than the cancer-producing effects that the smoke from the marijuana plant may have on the lungs and air passages of the individual.

Persons who use marijuana claim that it gives them a relaxed feeling. It separates them from the pressures of living. Some individuals claim that they experience sensual and pleasurable feelings toward other people. They find that the use of this plant helps them to socialize better.

Police officers should clearly understand that individuals under the influence of marijuana have a reduced ability for driving automobiles, for productive study, and for the making of critical decisions. Individuals under the influence of marijuana may converse profusely; however, they do not converse intelligently. Finally, it seems clear that fine motor control on the part of individuals under the influence of marijuana is reduced.

There are certain reported physiological effects of the drug marijuana on human behavioral patterns. For example, there seems to be a time and space distortion. Individuals under the influence of this chemical tend to have tunnel vision (decreased peripheral vision.) Certain sense perceptions seem to be increased—specifically, the senses of sound, taste, and feeling (tactile).

Many individuals under the influence of marijuana find difficulty in coordinating their movements. Some show frank hallucinations. Virtually all individuals under the influence have an increased appetite and show a reddening of the eyes due to inflammation and irritation of the wet tissues of the eye. The harsh cough that often accompanies marijuana smoking is the result of irritating products of burning plant material.

There are possible negative effects of using marijuana that should be kept in mind. Many individuals exhibit confusion, anxiety, panic, and paranoia. A large number of users show impairment of judgment or of memory. In some instances, individuals report a lessening of inhibitions.

The level of intoxication after taking marijuana by inhalation starts out at zero at the time of beginning the experience. After using whatever amount of marijuana is available, the individual will probably experience a maximum effect about an hour and a half after taking the final dose.   The effect then wears off so that, ordinarily, by the end of four hours after the individual has taken the drug, he has returned to his baseline or nonintoxicated level. Various kinds of stress may bring about the immediate termination of the so-called "high" that comes from using marijuana: some event like an arrest or an accident seems to have an instant sobering effect on the user.   Ordinarily, during the period when the drug is affecting the user, the individual is relaxed, passive, and shows a certain amount of drowsiness.

Stimulants

Stimulants are a group of chemicals that act on certain parts of the brain and spinal cord to increase the response of the body to various stimuli.   A good example of a chemical stimulant is amphetamine.   This chemical is a stimulant for the central nervous system.   It is a legally used drug and is marketed under such names as Dexedrine®, Benzedrine®, and other similar commercial titles. There is a related compound called methamphetamine or methadrine.

Stimulants have been used by physicians for a long time.   Recently these chemicals have been abused more and more by the general public.   A committee on alcoholism and addiction pointed out that in 1966, there were sufficient tablets of amphetamine available in the United States to give every person between twenty-five to fifty doses of amphetamine.

These drugs are abused by every group in our society.   They are abused by truck drivers, housewives, students, and businessmen.   There is no truth to the popular view that abusers of stimulants are dropouts with long dirty hair, bare feet, and smelly clothing.   This kind of view does little to help us understand the problem of abuse of stimulants.

Amphetamines bring about stimulation of the central nervous system all the way from the higher portions of the brain down through the spinal cord.   Ordinarily the brain is the primary location where stimulation takes place.   The effect of amphetamines is to cause an intense prolonged stimulation, which then is followed by a deep depression.

Mood, mental processes, and overall sensations seem to be elevated or magnified. Overdose with amphetamines causes strange and weird behavior. The victim becomes aggressive, he may have hallucinations, and he may go into convulsions. The depression stage that follows the metabolizing of the drug by the body is referred to as *the crash* or *crashing*. The complete exhaustion follows inevitably the long-time excessive activity brought about by the amphetamines. The heart responds to this stimulated activity by increasing its rate and its output. The blood vessels surrounding the heart and supplying the heart muscle with blood for its action are dilated more than usual as a result of the stimulating action of amphetamines.

Ronaghan (1972) points out that "constriction of blood vessels results in elevation of blood pressure. This is a secondary reaction to stimulation of the vasomotor centers in the brain." He goes on to explain "that abusers of stimulants are prone to physical changes in arteries. They develop necrotizing angiitis, a syndrome similar to periarteritis nodosa which has a high incidence of mortality . . . The necrotizing angiitis may be produced by oral ingestion as well as by intravenous injection of amphetamines."

Loss of appetite frequently accompanies the use of amphetamines. In fact, it is this reaction to amphetamines that resulted in their use by many physicians in weight-reduction programs. Some damage to the blood vessels and the kidneys has been reported. Hepatitis has been observed among abusers of stimulants, especially those who inject amphetamines. This is not a direct effect of the amphetamine but results from the sharing of dirty injection equipment.

GENERAL EFFECTS. The general effects of abuse of amphetamines include loss of appetite and insomnia. Individuals who chronically take moderate amounts of amphetamines often develop what is called *acute toxic psychosis*. This condition often requires hospitalization over a long period of time. There is strong and well documented evidence that points to the conclusion that abusers of amphetamines are more likely to engage in acts of violence then are nonabusers. Individuals who are under the influence of amphetamines tend to show what is called *compulsive behavior*. Compulsive behavior may be useful, but it also may be destructive.

DEATH.   Death may be a secondary development to the abuse of amphetamines. Death may result from malnutrition because of loss of appetite. It may result from the hepatitis brought about by the use and sharing of dirty injection equipment. Congestion of the blood vessels in the lungs and brain can result in death. Suicide is an important cause of death among abusers of amphetamines simply because of the psychosis that results from the abuse. It is known that cardiovascular diseases referred to above can bring death. Finally, an assortment of infections associated secondarily with the abuse of amphetamines also must be recognized as a cause of death in this group of drug abusers.

There seems to be no valid use outside the medical field for amphetamines or methamphetamines.

Cocaine

Another stimulant that has become popular among the "jet set" is cocaine. For some reason that makes no scientific sense, cocaine is classed as a narcotic under the Harrison Narcotic Act. Biologically, cocaine is not a narcotic, but a stimulant for the central nervous system. Its biological effects on the body are similar to amphetamine or to methamphetamine.

There is no evidence that cocaine is physiologically addicting. However, there are claims that it is psychologically addicting. Case histories are available that show that prolonged regular use of cocaine may cause a social behavior best described as weird. Usually the morphine-type addict avoids the cocaine user simply because of the individual's tendency toward unpredictable behavior.

EFFECTS.   There are a number of clearly defined effects of the abuse of cocaine. Among these is excessive irritability of the central nervous system. This can result in convulsions and death. Cocaine users show a loss of appetite much like that found among abusers of amphetamines. Gastrointestinal upsets are common. The stimulating phase of cocaine use is always followed by a severe depression, which can result in suicide and other destructive acts. Cocaine is characterized by causing unpredictable behavior that seems to bear no relationship to the environment surrounding the abuser. Acts of violence, assaults, and paranoid psychosis all result from cocaine abuse. There seems to be reasonable evidence that psychological addiction to cocaine is a fact. Many individuals who are psychologically addicted to cocaine commit suicide when the chemical is taken away from them.

COCAINE HAZARDS. Deaths from abuse of cocaine are known to occur; Cocaine is not an absolutely safe drug of abuse. Indeed, the numbers of accidental deaths from cocaine seem to be increasing in North America, especially among young, white males having a record of drug abuse (Finkle and McCloskey, 1978). There is a popular false belief among drug abusers that inhaling cocaine is a completely safe route of self-administration. Nasal insufflation (sniffing) as a route of administration was known to have been involved in 8 deaths directly attributable to cocaine abuse. Blood concentration of cocaine in these corpses was high, 2.8 to 5.9 μg of cocaine per ml of blood. Blood levels of cocaine in fatalities, caused by abuse of the drug are found to be, as a rule, less than 9.0 μg/ml of blood.

Blood should be taken, in preference to any other body tissue or fluid, in all death cases where cocaine is suspected to have been involved.

Analytical methods for cocaine are adequate, and most analytical laboratories can carry out competent quantitative analyses for the drug. With a 5 ml sample of blood, sensitivities of about 1.0 to 2.0 μg/ml of blood should be obtained.

Polydrug Use

As pointed out elsewhere in this book, polydrug use is now becoming more common than the abuse of a single drug. In keeping with this general tendency, more and more abusers of cocaine combine it with heroin to produce a mixture called the A-bomb or the atomic bomb cocktail. The heroin in the mixture serves to lengthen the duration of the feeling of ecstasy brought about by the cocaine. Also, the heroin seems to ease or quiet the crash or annoying depression that usually and ordinarily occurs after the effects of cocaine wear off.

Cocaine is used importantly as a local anesthetic. As cocaine in this use is not injected but applied to a surface, it is called a topical anesthetic. There are no valid nonmedical uses for cocaine.

Ronaghan (1972) concludes that "Abusers develop a strong psychological addiction to this chemical. When combined with heroin they run the added risk of a physiological addiction due to the addicting properties of heroin."

Methamphetamine

This chemical is a central nervous system stimulant. It is sometimes referred to as *speed*. The average dose of methamphetamine when used medically is between 5 and 15 mg per individual. Abusers of this drug, when they are on what is called a *speed binge,* may use anywhere from 1 to 15 gm of methamphetamine per day. The hard user may repeatedly inject himself with this drug from 2 to 10 times a day. Many of these individuals go through this same binge cycle again and again. Each time they inject methamphetamine rapidly, they get what is called a *flash* or a *body orgasm*. The abuser of this drug may persist in the "high" state for several days. Between injections or hits, the abuser experiences euphoria; he is hyperactive and readily excited by virtually any environmental change. This condition may last for 5 days, during which time the abuser does not sleep and rarely, if ever, takes food. Eventually, this high state wears off, and the individual discontinues the activity as a result of fatigue, confusion, paranoia, or panic or because the usual amount of the drug no longer brings on the desired effect.

While the drug is acting on the victim, the latter is hyperexcitable; this stage is followed by one of extreme exhaustion. During the exhaustion stage, the abuser may sleep from 24 to 48 hours without a break. When he does awaken, he shows psychological depression in many instances, he may be extremely hungry, or he may move into a long-term subacute stage of extreme physiological depression. This depression may be so severe and so unpleasant for the user that he starts another binge. In all too many instances, the depression problem is settled by suicide.

Adverse effects of this drug have been clearly demonstrated time and again, in one place after another where users operate. During the high stage, there is a major break with reality—what is known as *toxic psychosis* may develop—and the individual may need to be treated in a hospital. Individuals have paranoid or even schizophrenic responses and the potential for suicide by users of this drug is extremely high. The drug tends to push the body beyond any reasonable mental or physical capabilities. The abuser, in order to maintain a high or to repeat a high to get himself out of a depression, is prone to overmedicate himself. During the period of the high, which is then followed by the depression stage, little effective social life is possible. Since the abuser shows fear and distrust for other persons, he readily alienates his friends, employers, and teachers.

The increased physical and psychological activity that the drug stimulates is carried out without judgment and consideration. Consequently, the actions of an individual under the influence of methamphetamine often are extremely hard to interpret by normal individuals. The subject shows signs of confusion, irritability, and hostility. Inevitably, such individuals come in conflict with the law and waste much energy and money in this activity.

Is methamphetamine physically addicting? It is possible to show, in some instances, physical dependence of an abuser on the drug. The tolerance potential is high. After one or two binges, the individual must then take enormous doses to bring on a similar high. In many cases, even doses that approach fatality cannot reinstitute a high after one or two binges. The psychological potential for dependence is high.

The drug is usually administered by vein, and consequently the flash, rush, or body orgasm occurs quickly. Then there is a prolonged stage of euphoria, or what is sometimes called an *action stage*. During this time, the individual shows increased motor ability and excitability, the hands show pronounced tremor, and the user is talkative, cannot sleep, perspires, and has no interest in food. This action phase is followed by the crash, when the effects of the drug wear off. During this time, one sees in the user what might be called an *acute anxiety reaction*. The user is anxious, nervous, and hyperexcitable. Psychotic reactions include breaks with reality. The exhaustion stage, as indicated previously, lasts from 24 to 48 hours. Deaths associated with this drug are in many instances suicidal or accidental. Combination of this drug with others can indeed become a lethal potion.

Damage. This drug, which is a favorite in the drug-abusing world, shows no evidence of producing behavioral or physical dependence in rhesus monkeys given the chemical under experimental conditions. Food and water intakes seem to be unmodified, a fact that suggests another look is needed at the use of such drugs for weight control in human beings.

Of grave concern is the fact that studies on the brains of rhesus monkeys given methamphetamine chronically for 5 to 6 months showed degeneration of the nerve cells (neurons) and of the support cells in the brain (glial cells). The livers in these drugged monkeys showed changes visible under the electron microscope: "A marked proliferation of the smooth endoplasmic reticulum." This latter phenomenon is postulated to be associated with the tolerance to methamphetamine known to be developed (Weiss and Laties, 1975).

Reported Pathology. A number of pathological responses to amphetamine abuse have been documented in the biomedical literature (Ronaghan, 1972). Necrotizing angiitis (tissue-destroying inflammation of the arteries) is known to occur and may be fatal. Renal artery aneurysm also is associated with some abusers. Paranoia and violence are seen after chronic mild abuse of amphetamines.

Death from secondary causes has been recorded: malnutrition, hepatitis, blood vessel congestion in lungs and brain, suicide caused by psychosis, various diseases of the circulatory system, and infections.

The paranoid-hallucinatory syndrome is reported in some abusers (Temkov et al., 1976).

Lysergic Acid Diethylamide (LSD-25)

This drug is a prime example of a psychomimetic chemical, a chemical that creates in the user many of the signs and symptoms of insanity. LSD-25 is sometimes referred to as a hallucinogen because of the capacity the drug has in very small amounts to cause strange visions and distortions of consciousness.

The usual dosage, which is adequate to cause the mental effects of this drug, is 100 to 250 μg. The substance is colorless, odorless, and tasteless. It dissolves readily in water. It is readily absorbed from the gastrointestinal tract when it is swallowed. Doses as small as 25 μg have been reported to cause adverse psychological effects in particularly susceptible persons.

What is the attraction of LSD-25 for human abuse? Abusers claim that the drug is mind-expanding and increases sensory awareness. Self-meaning is amplified. The drug is supposed to make one "real." Some artists even claim that use of the drug increases creativity. Interestingly enough, none of these effects has ever been demonstrated in a quantitative way. The exponents of the creativity factor have never (as far as the written record is concerned) demonstrated this increased creativity as a result of taking the drug or in their own production of art or literary classics.

There is a latent period of between 30 and 40 minutes after swallowing an average dose. Some of the physiological responses to doses of LSD include dilation of the pupils, a slight rapid increase in blood pressure, and sometimes an increased pulse rate. Unpleasant responses have also been reported as a result of swallowing LSD-25. These include nausea, vomiting, sweating, chills, flushes, tingling sensations, tremors, dry mouth, irregularity of breathing, distortion of vision, and an increase body temperature. Whether all these signs and symptoms are properly attributed to the drug is questionable. The setting, the anticipation, and the apprehensions may all go into bringing about some of these peculiar physiological responses.

There are certain psychological reactions to LSD. One of the major reactions is a deep-seated and overwhelming anxiety. Individuals have a sense of depersonalization and express loss of their own body image. Perceptions are changed. In many instances, colors seem brighter, and sounds seem clearer.

In my own case during an experimental exposure to this agent, the anxiety factor was so overwhelming as to preclude my taking this drug ever again. I felt that I was approaching a cliff and that I would inevitably go over that cliff and be lost. My fall over the cliff was to be in slow motion. The strange aspect of this picture was that I felt I was looking down from above on myself in this problem. At times, I actually was able to hear colors and see certain sounds. At no time did I ever experience hallucinations. There is strong evidence that what hallucinations have been reported are actually pseudohallucinations.

The sense of time is frequently disrupted, with a merging and mixing of past, present, and future. In some cases, these experiences are so disrupting that the victim goes into a panic.

Despite the fact that there are claims for the mind-expanding action of this agent, in general, intellectual functions are harmed. There is an impairment of value judgment and learning functions; confusion results. In most cases, there is a bizarre association of thoughts. Thinking may be expanded, but it becomes so loose as to break into pieces. Individuals under the influence of this drug do not lose consciousness; they remember most of what went on. In several subjects that came to my attention experimentally, suspiciousness and hostility developed. In some instances are what is known as *flashbacks*. For some reason or other, individuals may go through this sad drug experience months later. They may have a recurrence of the acute reaction. These flashbacks, plus rethinking the acute reaction, sometimes can lead to long-term depression. It has been suggested that inadvertent suicide resulted in some cases from exposure to this drug. The documentation of these suicides is not adequate.

In individuals who are already disturbed or are on the borderline of some form of mental disability, the LSD experience can be devastatingly harmful. Such individuals may go into a long-term schizophrenic reaction. They may enter a long-term depression, which is punctuated by periodic reactions of panic. Flashbacks seem to be more common in the borderline cases than in the presumably normal user or abuser.

There is no evidence whatsoever of brain damage from this drug. The reported persistent changes in brain wave pattern of the chronic users of this drug are open to various interpretations. The factual existence of these persistent alterations is not well established.

The drug is not particularly popular among abusers, probably because of reports that chromosomes in the white blood cells of certain users showed modifications attributed to the LSD-25, although the basic laboratory studies that led to the publication of this report are of questionable validity. In the meantime, there is no documented demonstration of any human birth defects that can be even remotely attributed to the use of LSD-25.

LSD-25 has a high potential for toleration, which develops quickly. Anyone who attempts to abuse the drug cannot do so more than about twice a week or twice in ten days because, after the second dose, the third and fourth doses, no matter how heavy, cannot bring on the reaction. There is no physical dependency. The question of psychological dependency has not been established. The interesting point of this drug is that there is no lethal dosage for man. In other words, no one has ever been killed as a result of a lethal dose of LSD being swallowed. The effective dose is so low that no abuser has ever even approached a dose that could be considered anywhere near lethal.

Barbiturates

Barbiturates are depressants. They are used extensively under prescription for helping persons with insomnia and aiding people who need to be sedated or tranquilized. The common forms in which the barbiturates are available are red-colored capsules that contain 100 mg of Seconal each; yellow-colored capsules that contain 100 mg of Nembutal each; and capsules that are blue and red containing Tuinal®, which consists of 50 mg of Amytal plus 50 mg of Nembutal to make a total of 100 mg of Tuinal.

The illicit drug trade refers to these different preparations as reds, yellows, blues, or blue and reds. Barbiturates are ordinarily taken by mouth, although they may at times be injected into a vein. However, it is not medically sensible to break open a capsule of one of the barbiturates, dissolve the contents in water, and then inject it without special buffering chemicals. The solution of the contents of these colored capsules results in a liquid that is extremely irritating to all living tissue. The pH value of such a solution is about 12, which indicates that the solution is extremely alkaline.

The dose needed to get the desired effect from barbiturates is between 50 and 100 mg. Tolerance develops, and it develops quickly. As an example, it takes only a few weeks of repeated doses for the development of a high to require as much as 400 to 1000 mg, whereas at the beginning of the abuse, only 50 to 100 mg were needed. The amount of barbiturate needed to bring unconsciousness also goes up as tolerance develops.

Why do some individuals abuse barbiturates? According to available information, abusers maintain that these drugs help them to relax, help them to "relate to others." They bring on a grumpy condition that seems to be similar to that following the intake of too much alcohol. Finally, some abusers say that their self-confidence is enhanced.

There are a number of reactions that are harmful to individuals who use these drugs. The acute reactions include confusion and stupor. Some individuals become belligerent after taking these drugs, just as some individuals become belligerent after using alcohol. Most show a lack of coordination. Overdoses are all too common, with death resulting from unconsciousness and depression of the breathing system of the body.

Individuals who are chronic or long-term abusers of barbiturates show irreversible brain damage. They may die of convulsions. Withdrawal symptoms are violent and frequently lead to death. In other words, the withdrawal syndrome associated with barbiturates is much more devastating than is the withdrawal syndrome associated with opium addiction.

The straightforward physiological effects of these drugs include depression of the cerebral portion of the brain, followed by classic stages of anesthesia. These start out with euphoria, or the feeling of a general high pleasant aspect. This is followed by an excitement stage, and finally stupor and actual sleep. If the dose is large enough, respiratory depression, unconsciousness, and death result. The so-called high with euphoria and relaxation occurs between 30 and 60 minutes and is over by 2 to 4 hours. Thereafter sleep results.

Overdosage is not uncommon with these drugs. Barbiturates are used in a large number of intentional suicides.

WITHDRAWAL. The withdrawal problem is a serious one. The fact of physical addiction to barbiturates is well established. Withdrawal brings on such abnormal responses as twitching of the muscles and surly and temperamental behavior; the hands show tremor. When the withdrawal is absolute, delirium and hallucinations result. The reaction is much like the DTs associated with alcohol withdrawal. Fever often accompanies the withdrawal from barbiturates. Death results after development of severe convulsions.

Withdrawal from barbiturate addiction must be done only in a hospital under rigid medical supervision. Withdrawal from barbiturates can be accomplished successfully, resulting in permanent cure of the addiction. It cannot be done by a cold turkey method. It cannot be done on one's own initiative. It must be carried out in a hospital under medical supervision.

Tranquilizers

Tranquilizers form a group of chemicals that were introduced into the United States in the early 1950s. They were primarily aimed at use by psychiatrists. Tranquilizers are used extensively in mental hospitals, especially with patients who previously had little chance for rehabilitation. By the use of tranquilizers, it has been possible to communicate with previously hopeless persons in custodial care at mental institutions.

As with most chemicals, these tranquilizers have been and are being abused by some elements in our society. The general effects of abuse of tranquilizers might be summarized as follows: Tolerance can develop so that individuals have to take ever-increasing doses in order to get the desired effect. Abusers tend to show a general lethargy disposing them to be less than effective in their work. Chronic users of tranquilizers show a flushed skin and chronic nasal congestion. Many of them develop postural hypotension, a condition in which standing in an upright position causes a blood pressure so low that the individual faints. In a lying down or even a sitting position, such individuals can carry on in a normal fashion. In a standing position, they are prone to fainting. Abusers of tranquilizers show an allergic skin rash in many instances. They are subject to depression and difficulties with walking, and they have vivid and often disturbing dreams. Of great concern is the fact that chronic use of tranquilizers may damage the blood. Chronic abusers often show jaundice or a generalized yellowish color of the skin; this sign indicates possible damage to the liver. Most tranquilizers have associated with them psychological addiction; a few tranquilizers cause physiological addiction.

Deaths from overdoses of tranquilizers are becoming more common. The cause of death is collapse of the breathing system of the body. In some instances, death may be accidental as a result of impaired judgment resulting from the action of the tranquilizer on the brain. Collapse of the respiratory system is almost inevitable if tranquilizers are used in conjunction with alcohol or barbiturates.

How Tranquilizers Act on the Body. Tranquilizers in general depress selectively certain important zones and pathways in the brain. Many drugs that depress the nervous system have an increased effect when they are used along with tranquilizers. Such drugs include opium and its derivatives, sedatives of all sorts, alcohol, and various anesthetic agents.

The hypothalamus, which is a key portion of the brain, is depressed by tranquilizers. This depressant action results in a slowing down of the basal metabolic rate of the body. The body temperature is decreased. There is increased drowsiness. The blood vessels of the body become less effective in controlling blood pressure. The vomiting center, which is located in the hypothalamus, is depressed. Indirectly, action on the hypothalamus may have an effect on the pituitary gland, which, of course, is the master gland of the body; such an effect could influence the normal balance of hormones in the body.

The heart rate is often decreased, primarily as a result of the psychic depression caused by the tranquilizers. The blood vessels in the outlying body areas tend to dilate. This action is especially pronounced in the shock that accompanies overdose of tranquilizers.

The respiratory or breathing system of the body is not affected when ordinary therapeutic doses are given. If massive doses are given, collapse of the respiratory system often occurs.

Jaundice is observed in some individuals who take tranquilizers over a long period of time. Tranquilizers taken in combination with a number of other drugs often cause damage of the liver. There are no recorded adverse effects on the kidney. However, under certain circumstances, the digestive system may be upset when tranquilizers are given. Reserpine, which is a tranquilizer that allays anxiety, is known to cause ulcers in the stomach and in the duodenum.

MEDICAL USES. There are important and valid uses of tranquilizers by physicians. Of primary importance is the use of these drugs in such behavioral conditions as schizophrenia, senile dementia, and general manic conditions. Tranquilizers are sometimes used under controlled conditions to alleviate acute alcoholism. When used judiciously, tranquilizers may help an alcoholic to pass through the withdrawal symptoms. Tranquilizers also are used medically to control nausea and vomiting. In the hospital, tranquilizers may be used along with various anesthetics. A number of tranquilizers are useful as chemicals that relax the muscles.

There seems to be no appropriate nonmedical use of tranquilizers.

Narcotics

Narcotics are chemicals that act primarily to depress the central nervous system. There are a large number of narcotics available to the medical profession, all of which are some form of chemical derivative of opium, the basic material found in the opium poppy. Opium itself is used medically as a treatment for stomach and intestinal difficulties. A solution of opium with some camphor added is sold as paragoric, which is also used for gastrointestinal difficulties.

Morphine is used widely by physicians to relieve pain. It is obtained by purifying opium and isolating morphine from the natural product. If the morphine is methylated, it results in codeine, which is an excellent pain reliever, especially dental pain.

Heroin was originally synthesized by German chemists in an attempt to produce a derivative of opium that was less addicting than morphine. Morphine, when combined with acetic acid, gives diacetyl morphine, the chemical name for heroin. Although heroin was designed to be less addicting than morphine, in fact it is much more addicting than is morphine. It is favored by drug abusers. Dionin is morphine combined with the organic ethyl group. There are a number of synthetic narcotics made in an attempt to improve on the basic qualities of morphine. Among these are metapon, Demerol®, (also known as Meperidine®, Isomipecaine®, Dolation®, and Pethidine®) as well as Methadone® (also named Adanon®, Amalone®, Dolophine®, and Amidon®).

Morphine, probably the most important drug available to a physician, is used as the reference standard for potency and effectiveness. Many physicians maintain that if they were isolated on a desert island with the responsibility for taking care of a group of castaways and the physician were allowed a single drug and no others, they would choose morphine. It is a safe drug. Given properly by a physician, it is an effective drug. The various synthetic forms of morphine and the derivatives vary from the basic morphine in several ways. For example, codeine has only 17 percent of the potency of morphine, whereas heroin is 10 times as potent as morphine; Dilaudid® is also 10 times as potent as morphine. Dionin has only 17 percent of the potency of morphine, whereas Metapon® is twice as potent as morphine. Demanol® has 50 percent of the potency of morphine, whereas methadone has about the same potency as morphine.

Morphine, as an example of this group of drugs known as narcotics, depresses the higher centers of the brain, beginning with the cerebral cortex. The routes for pain from various parts of the body to the cortex of the brain are interrupted by morphine. Given morphine for pain, the subject slowly loses consciousness of a response to pain. Motor pathways, that is, the pathways that control voluntary movement, are depressed by large doses of morphine. With very large doses, unconsciousness results, the hypo-thalamus of the brain is depressed, and thus the body temperature tends to decrease when morphine is given.

The medulla is also depressed. Consequently, the heart rate and the rate of breathing decreases in patients under the influence of morphine. Interestingly enough, the vomiting center in the brain is stimulated and made more sensitive in the morphine-treated patient. Quite often the patient given morphine for the first time becomes nauseated and vomits. On the other hand, the cough center is depressed; thus, some cough medicines have co-deine added in order to suppress excessive coughing that may be weakening a patient. In general, the various vegetative functions of the body are depressed. One of the characteristics of morphine derivatives is that they cause constipation. Most heroin addicts are chronically constipated and must take unusual means to re-lieve that situation.

Generally, morphine and its derivatives do not cause perma-nent and major damage to any organ system in the body. In this respect, morphine is different than alcohol, tobacco smoke, amphetamines, or other drugs of abuse. The usual damage from morphine addiction results from secondary diseases caused by un-sanitary and filthy conditions associated with the abuse. There is one caution that should be kept in mind: Morphine and its de-rivatives all pass through the placental barrier and get into the growing fetus. This condition is of concern to pregnant women who are morphine addicts during their pregnancy. Almost in-variably the child of an addicted mother is born as an addict. Such addicted newborn infants must have special treatment in order for them to survive.

There is no known nonmedical use for narcotics.

Heroin

Heroin is an excellent example of the opium class of drugs. Historically, opium and its many derivatives have been abused by human beings for as long as opium was available to mankind. Heroin itself is morphine that has been treated with acetic acid, sometimes referred to as acetylated morphine. The drug heroin is ordinarily administered by vein, but it may be inhaled or administered by injecting under the skin. If swallowed, it is active.

One of the physiological effects of heroin administration is mild depression of the cerebrum. An interesting point, however, is that there is absolutely no interference with complex reasoning, judgment, or coordination. This point must be clearly remembered when evaluating the threat of heroin addiction to human society. When taken into the body, heroin is an excellent pain killer. It suppresses coughs. It also inhibits the activity of the intestine and of the bladder. The pupils of the eyes are constricted after taking heroin. There is no decrease in appetite as a result of the heroin intake, nor is there any decrease in sex interest or sex performance as a result of doses of heroin.

Why do addicts take heroin? According to all available reports, the "high" associated with the administration by vein of heroin is supposed to be the most intense euphoria known. It is said by some to be more satisfying than sex and reportedly lasts longer. The individual gets a feeling of floating in space at complete peace with the entire world. His needs are restricted to heroin; he needs nothing else. If less heroin than that needed to produce a high is taken, it serves as an ideal tranquilizer. Individuals under the influence of such doses have no cares or worries in the world. They live in a sea of tranquility.

Tolerance to heroin develops quickly. Consequently, with repeated usage, the amount needed to bring on the pleasurable effects increases dramatically. Physical addiction to heroin develops only if the abuser uses the drug consistently for several consecutive days. Weekenders who play around with heroin for years, but only intermittently, do so without showing any signs of physical addiction.

Withdrawal symptoms are startling and include runny nose, sweating and chills, pains in the joints and muscles, nausea, vomiting, and diarrhea. The process is not ordinarily fatal, as with barbiturate withdrawal. The "cold turkey" process is effective for withdrawal and poses no unacceptable hazard to the victim.

Indications of Poisoning at Autopsy

Drug Tablets in the Stomach

The condition of a drug tablet in the stomach can be readily observed during an autopsy. One study of the dissolution of tablets in the stomach showed that 11 percent of persons who lived from 6 hours to 7 days after taking a drug in tablet form exhibited undissolved tablets in the stomach at autopsy; 42 percent had visible granules of the preparation in the stomach under the same conditions; 38 percent gave positive qualitative results for the drug in the stomach contents, even in persons living 7 days after taking the overdose by mouth (Watanabe, 1968). The results of such a study demonstrate that frequently tablets of a drug or other poison persist in the stomach for days in the unconscious individuals. Consequently, there is every reason to wash out the stomach of a drug overdose victim even if the overdose were ingested a number of days previously.

In all poisoning fatalities that result from swallowing the toxic agent, the stomach contents must be collected at autopsy for possible identification of the toxic agent (or agents) ingested. The possibility of successful identification is high.

Analytical Methods

Reid (1976) recently published a technically excellent monograph on the analysis of body fluids for drugs and other compounds occurring in minute amounts.

Drugs are Poisons

Drugs are poisons and hence must under all circumstances be treated with respect and caution (Gouveia et al, 1976). Adverse reactions to drugs administered therapeutically by physicians, in the hospital and out of the hospital, are not uncommon. Indeed, some experts are surprised that adverse reactions are not more frequent in the light of such surveys as one covering the average number of drugs found in hospitalized patients who had been under care for at least three days; in the blood of these hospitalized patients there was an average of twenty-four distinct drug species.

A Boston Collaborative Drug Surveillance report suggests that of all acute drug exposures, nearly 6 percent involve adverse reactions. The most frequent complaints (in descending order of frequency) are nausea, drowsiness, diarrhea, vomiting, rash, irregularities of heartbeat, itching, trouble at the site of injection, increase in blood potassium, and fever. Of the reactions 60 percent came on gradually; the balance developed suddenly. Another way of saying this is that 40 percent of the adverse reactions occurred suddenly; these are the kind that can lead to death and the need for police investigation of the episode. These cases, when death supervenes, are clearly within the purview of the coroner or medical investigator. Fortunately, only about 10 percent of the reactions are classified as *serious* or *severe*. Of all adverse reactions, 75 percent cleared up within a week.

What kind of drugs most frequently cause trouble for the patient? The results of a survey made in Scotland between 1967 and 1974 help to answer the question (Table 4-I).

Table 4-I
ADVERSE REACTIONS TO DRUGS
SCOTLAND, 1967-1974

Kind of Drug (Target of Drug)	Number of Adverse Reactions
Anti-infection	238
Nervous system	237
Heart and blood vessels	128
Endocrine-metabolic	61
Cellular poison and nutritional	40
Diagnostic agents	13
Digestive tract	13
Skin preparations	1

One must be extremely cautious in the interpretation of data such as these. For example, "A large percentage of patients with life-threatening drug reactions go to teaching hospitals and it is not appropriate to extrapolate the findings from these hospitals to the total hospital universe" (Francke, 1974). Koch-Weser (1974) maintains that, "Estimates of lethal drug reactions based on extrapolations of their apparent prevalence on acute medical teaching services to the total number of hospital admissions in the United States are grossly misleading."

Polydrug Abuse

The good old days when drug abusers zeroed in on a single chemical in order to get their kicks are no more. Polydrug (poly meaning *many* or *more than one)* abuse is now the style. Depressants and stimulants are mixed; hallucinogens and tranquilizers are taken together. Alcohol seems to serve as a common matrix drug used with one or more others at the same time (Geldmacher et al., 1976). The unique hazards of drug interactions when several kinds are given simultaneously to a human being are well documented (Morselli et al, 1974). "It has been known for quite some time that the combination of two or more drugs often produces therapeutic or toxic results which may be quite different than what would be expected knowing the pharmacological action of each of the single compounds involved."

The details of only some mechanisms of drug interaction are known. The problem of polydrug use is complex, and our state of knowledge gives little support for predicting either acute or long-term effects of such practice on the abusers. It is certain, however, that polydrug abuse poses additional and as yet not clearly outlined hazards to the abusers.

Investigators working on poisoning cases should be keenly aware of the possibility that they may be facing a death or severe injury resulting from the ingestion of more than a single drug by the victim (Morselli et al., 1974).

In polydrug-alcohol deaths, blood alcohol levels of 0.041 to 0.28% are reported. These values are lower than in deaths caused by alcohol alone (Geldmacher et al, 1976). Survival time is about four hours or less.

Results of an investigation on the presence of ethanol in drug-intoxicated persons brought to hospital emergency rooms have been reported. In addition to other toxicologic analyses, specimens of blood, urine, and gastric content were analyzed for the presence of ethanol. Based on a request by the physician for analysis of drugs other than ethanol in 183 specimens, 34 were found to be positive for ethanol. Thus, it is concluded that the presence of ethanol in drug-intoxicated persons is often overlooked. Clinical recognition of ethanol intoxication in attempted suicide and accidental poisoning cases were also reported. It is suggested that all patients brought to the hospital with a diagnosis of drug intoxication should have a quantitative blood ethanol analysis in addition to analyses for other drugs (Hirsch and others, 1973).

Table 4-II summarizes the effects on man of polydrug abuse.

Table 4-II

THE TOXIC EFFECTS OF ALCOHOL PLUS VARIOUS MEDICATIONS*

Alcohol Plus	*Effect*
Antihistamines	Depression, drowsiness.
Aspirin	Bleeding in digestive tract.
Narcotics	Depression of brain centers; possible stoppage of breathing.
Painkillers	Irritation of digestive tract; bleeding possible.
Antabuse®	Increased breathing rate, vomiting, drowsiness.
High blood pressure control drugs	Greater effect. Fainting.
Anticoagulants by mouth	Greater effect at first. Chronic alcoholics show less effect.
Antidiabetic drugs by mouth	Much like Antabuse. Lessened effect on diabetes.
Antibiotics	Much like Antabuse.
Sedatives (barbiturates) and tranquilizers (Valium®, etc.)	Greater depression of brain and spinal cord; readily lethal.

*(Stockton, 1978)

Animal Data and Human Reactions

More and more toxicologists are persuaded that toxic effects of drugs and other chemicals in man are not generally predictable from animal studies (Wolstenholme and Porter, 1967). The results of animal tests are usually of limited value when the data are extrapolated to man; often animal data confuses and misleads with respect to what happens in man. "Unexpected toxic effects that do not depend on dosage, occur only occasionally in man, and are not predictable from animal studies are the greatest concern of the clinicians." Strangely enough, this basic understanding now held so widely by experts on poisonings in man is flagrantly ignored by federal agencies who make rules and regulations about the safety and effectiveness of a multitude of chemicals, drugs, and chemical formulations used for various purposes in the United States.

Sudden Death in Addicts

Abusers of opium derivatives, especially if these compounds are injected by the addict, are prone to sudden deaths that are still not fully explained. In many instances, these deaths occur while the drug is actually being injected. Most investigating officers are familiar with the picture of a dead addict, foam about his mouth and nose, the hypodermis needle still in place in a vein.

Johnston and co-workers (1969) of the Armed Forces Institute of Pathology have prepared a detailed study of the toxicological aspects of these deaths. Their study is based on the rather complete records of thirty addicts who died suddenly following the injection by vein of a narcotic. The amount of morphine in the kidneys, as revealed by chemical analysis (Goldbaum and Williams, 1968), is a useful sign of death following an injection of a narcotic. After such deaths, small amounts of morphine can be detected in bile and urine of the victims, "but the concentration was not a good indicator of recent intravenous injection" (Johnston et al., 1969).

In all victims who had died suddenly as a result of intervenous narcotism, the kidneys contained 0.2 mg of morphine or more per 100 gm of kidney tissue. Addicts who had died of other causes showed lower amounts of morphine in the kidneys. An interesting case comes to mind of a twenty-one-year-old male addict who had given himself an intravenous injection of heroin. He then attempted to steal additional narcotics from a companion, who killed him instantly with a shot through the chest. The victim had a concentration of 0.15 mg morphine per 100 gm of tissue in the kidneys, a value in keeping with the recent intravenous injection, although the sudden death in this case was not caused by the narcotic.

In most addicts, foreign materials are found in various tissues of the body. Lesions (pathological changes in any tissue of the body) are caused early by these foreign materials. Lung tissue is probably the best to examine for revealing foreign material introduced into the body along with the narcotic. Careful examination of the lungs under the microscope using polarized light should be a routine procedure in any complete postmortem examination of an addict's remains. Table 4-III shows the kinds of foreign materials to expect in lung tissue from addicts.

Table 4-III
FOREIGN MATERIAL FOUND IN LUNG TISSUE OF ADDICTS

Foreign Material Observed	*Percent of Addicts*
Any intravascular foreign material	78
Talc crystals	56
Embolic cotton fibers	11
Carbon particles	6
Unidentified	6

Some Conclusions

Hepatitis is secondary to narcotic abuse and results primarily from using and sharing filthy injecting gear, as well as living under foul conditions and eating disgusting food. Secondary infections seen in addicts result from the same sources as the hepatitis.

Malnourishment usually is an aspect of narcotic addiction for two main reasons:

1. The addict loses interest in food.
2. Because morphine and its derivatives are so costly on the illegal market, most of the addict's resources must be used to purchase his favorite drug; little money, if any, is left for food.

Finally, the following signs seen in morphine addicts are directly related to the abused drug: constipation, sweating and flushed skin, decrease in body temperature, shock, and coma.

Death can and does result from an overdose of the drug abused,

Table 4-IV

MINIMUM LETHAL DOSE OF REPRESENTATIVE DRUGS OF ABUSE

Drug	Minimum Lethal Dose
Amphetamine	1 gm
Amytal®	2 gm
Butobarbitone	2 gm
Chloral hydrate	2 gm
Cocaine	500 mg
Codeine	800 mg
Meprobamate (Miltown®)	50 gm
Morphine	200 mg
Nalorphine	200 mg
Nembutal®	2 gm
Dilaudid®	100 mg
Doriden®	5 gm
Ethyl alcohol	400 mg
Ethyl morphine	500 mg
Librium®	50 gm
Seconal®	2 gm

1 gram is equal to 1/28 of an ounce.

as a result of damage to the liver from secondary causes, because of an accident that happens usually as a result of the addict's defective judgment, or as the result of a possible host of secondary infections, among which are malaria, tetanus, endocarditis, and syphilis.

Withdrawal signs and symptoms are harsh but not usually fatal. Nevertheless, withdrawal from narcotic addiction should take place under formal, careful medical supervision.

Summary

In order to summarize information about the more commonly abused drugs, listed below are representative psychotropic drugs in various categories (Usdin and Efron, 1972). Usdin and Efron include extensive references to assay methods.*

*i.v. — intravenously   i.g. — intragastrically
 i.p. — intraperitoneally   i.m. — intramuscularly
 s.c. — subcutaneously   b.i.d — twice a day
 p.o. — by mouth   t.i.d. — three times a day

Stimulants

(–) **Cocaine**

2β-Carbomethoxy-3β-benzoxytropane.

Anina, benzoylmethylecgonine, Bernice, Bernies, Burese, "C" Carrie, Cecil, cholly coke, Corine, ecgonine methylester benzoate, dust, Eritroxilina, Erytroxylin, flake, girl, gold dust, happy dust, Kokain, Kokan, Kokayeen, Neurocaine, snow, star dust.

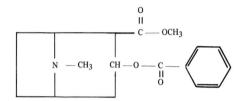

LD$_{50}$:   17.5 mg/kg/i.v./rats

Methamphetamin (e)

N,α-Dimethylphenethylamine hydrochloride.

A 884, Amdram (Dram), Amedrine (Brazil), Amphedroxyn® (Lilly), Apamine (Stillco), bombita, businessman's trip, Corvitin, Daropervamin, Deaoxo-5, Deofed (Drug Prod.), deoxyephedrine, Depoxin, Desamin(e) (Starr), Desfedran (Abbott, Chile), Desfedrin® (Abbott, Argentina), desossiefedrina, Des-Oxa-D (Walker), Desoxedrine (Testagar), Desoxin, Desoxo-5 (Sut. & Case), desoxyephedrin(e), Desoxyfed®, Desoxyn(e)® (Abbott), Desoxyphed, Destim®, Desyphed (Sterl-Win.), Desyphen, Detrex (Mallard), Dexophrine, Dexosyn, Dexoval® (Vale), Dexstim (Central), DOE® (Breon, Tilden Yates), Dopidrin, Doxephin, Doxephrin®, Doxyfed (Raymer), Drinalfa® (Squibb), Effroxine, Efroxine® (Maltbie, Wallace & Tiernan, Strasen), Estimulex, Eufodrin, Eufodrinal, Euphodrin, Euphodrinal, 914F, Fenyprin, Gerobit® (Berot), Gerovit, Heropon, Hiropon®, Isophan, Isophen® (Knoll), Kemodrin, Lanazine (Lannett), Levetamin, Madrine® (Langley), Mepho-d (Natl. Drug), metamfetamin(a), Metamina, Metamine, metamphetamin, Metamsustac (Pharmax), Metanfetamina, Methamphin (Rorer), Methedrinal, Methedrine® (Bur. Well., Brunnengraber), Methoxyn (Kenny), methylamphetamine(e),

Methylbenzedrin, Methylisamin, Methylisomin, Methylisomyn®, Methylpropamine, Miller-Drine (Miller), Neodrin(e), Neopharmedrine, Noradrin, Normadrine (Van Pelt & Brown), Norodin (Endo), Norodrin, Oxydess (Chimedic), Oxydrene, Oxydrin (Grant), Oxyfed (Cole), Pervitin® (SKF, Zilliken, Temmler, U.S.S.R.), Phedoxe (Elder), Phedrisox (Ascher), Philopon, Pisichergina, Premodrin (Premo), Psichergina, Psicopan, Psiquergina, Psychergine, Psykoton, Semoxydrine® (Massengill), Soxysympamine®, speed, Stimdex (Ulmer), Stimulex, Syndrox® (McNeill), Tonedrin, Tonedron®, Vonedrin(e). [Tartrate: Adipex® (Lemmon), Obesin (Zori).] [L isomer: Anahist (Anadrax-Wirkstoff); methylisonym.]

LD$_{50}$: 70 mg/kg/i.p./mice; for D isomer: 15 mg/kg/i.p./mice; 9.4 mg/kg/i.v./mice; for L isomer: 82 mg/kg/i.p./mice; 33 mg/kg/i.v./mice; 30 mg/kg/s.c./rats; 10 mg/kg/p.o./dogs; 2.7 mg/kg/i.v./dogs; 180 mg/kg/s.c./mice; 25 mg/kg/i.p./rats; 50 mg/kg/s.c./cats.

Action: Sedative (1240); hypnotic at large dose i.v.; sedative and anorectic.

Human Dose: Hypnotic dose: 40-60 mg/i.v.; sedative dose: 2.5-5 mg/b.i.d.-t.i.d.; 10-15 mg/i.v./b.i.d.; 15-30 mg/i.m./b.i.d; 2.5-10 mg daily; anorectic dose: 10-15 mg.

Depressants

Δ⁹-THC

6,6,9-Trimethyl-3-pentyl-7,8,9,10-tetrahydro-6H-dibenzo[b,d]pyran-1-ol.

(−)-Δ⁹-*trans*-Tetrahydrocannabinol, Δ¹-THC (monoterpenoid numbering).

LD$_{50}$: >1000 mg/kg/p.o./mice; >1000 mg/kg/i.p./mice; 1000-5000 mg/kg/i.p./mice; 29 mg/kg/i.v./rats; 373 mg/kg/i.p./rats; 666 mg/kg/i.g./rats; 42 mg/kg/i.v./mice; 454 mg/kg/i.p./mice; 482 mg/kg/i.g./mice.

Action: Hypnotic (450) ; hypnotic (in an.) .

Human Dose: 50-200 μg/kg/p.o.; 24-50 μg/kg/smoked.

Secobarbital

Sodium 5-allyl-5-(1-methylbutyl)barbiturate.

Barbosec, Biplinal®, Evronal, Hypotrol, Immenoctal®, Imesonal®, quinalbarbitone sodium, Quinalspan®, Seco 8 (Fleming), secobarbitone, Seconal® (Lilly) , Sedutain®, Seotal®, Trisomnin.

Action: Short-acting sedative; hypnotic.

Human Dose: 50-200 mg.

Pentobarbital

Sodium 5-ethyl-5-(1-methylbutyl)barbiturate.

Barpental®, Continal® (Teva) , Embutal®, Ethaminal, Euthatal®, Mebubarbital, Mebumal Sodium®, Mintal (Japan) , Nembutal® (Abbott) , Pentone®, pentobarbitone sodium, Pentothal®, Pentyl®, Rivadorn, Sagatal®, Sopental®, Sotyl®. [Calcium salt: Repocal®.]

LD$_{50}$: 130 mg/kg/i.p./mice; 280 mg/kg/p.o./mice; 33 mg/kg/p.o./newborn rats; 200 mg/kg/p.o./adult rats; 1 mg/kg/s.c./newborn mice; 30 mg/kg/s.c./adult mice.

Action: Sedative; short-acting hypnotic; anticonvulsant.

Human Dose: 30-300 mg/p.o.

Phenobarbital

5-Ethyl-5-phenylbarbituric acid.

Adonal (Vicario), Agrypnal® (eggo), Amylofene, Aphenylbarbit (Streuli), Aphenyletten (Streuli), Austrominal (Berger), Barbenyl®, Barbinal (Pharmacia-Denmark), Barbiphenyl®, Barbipil®, Barbita, Barbivis, Blu-phen, Cratecil®, Dormiral® (Heisler), Doscalun, Duneryl, Epidorm (Switzerland), Eskabarb® (SKF), Etilfen®, Euneryl®, Fenemal (Sweden), fenobarbital, Gardenal® (Specia, Rhone-Poulenc, M & B), Gardepanyl® (Gomennol), Helional (St. Veit), Hypnogen (Fragner), Hypnoltol(on) (Steiger), Leonal (Leo-Germany), Lepinal (Germany), Liquital, Liquital, Lixophen, Lubergal® (Braun & Herberg), Lubrokal® (Albert), Luminal® (Sterl-Win., Bayer, E. Merck), Neurobarb®, Noptil®, Numol, Nunol®, Phenaemal (Woelm), Phenemal, Phenemalum (Woelm), Phenobal®, phenobarbitone, Phenobarbyl (Synochem), Phenolurio, Phenomet, Phenonyl®, Phenyral® (Apogepha), Phob, Seda-Tablinen (Sanorania), Somonal®, Stental (Robins), Teolaxin, Teoloxin, Theoloxin, Triphenatol, Versomnal (France).

LD_{50}:   340 mg/kg/i.p./mice; 660 mg/kg/p.o./rats; 168 mg/ kg/p.o./mice; ca. 300 mg/kg/p.o./mice; 66 mg/kg/p.o./newborn rats; 162 mg/kg/p.o./adult rats.

Action: Hypnotic; long-acting sedative; anticonvulsant.

Human Dose: 15-100 mg.

Hallucinogens

Lysergic Acid Diethylamide

9,10-Didehydro-*N*,*N*-diethyl-6-methyl-ergoline-8β-carboxamide.

Acid, cubes, Delysid® (Sandoz), *N*,*N*-diethyl lysergamide, heavenly blue, LSD, LSD-25® (Sandoz), Lysergamid (Spofa), Lysergid(e), Lysergsäuere Diaethylamid®, Lysergäure Diethylamid®, pearly gates, royal blue, wedding bells.

LD_{50}:   46 mg/kg/i.v./mice; 16.5 mg/kg/i.v./rats; 0.3 mg/kg/ i.v./rabbits; 65 mg/kg/i.v./mice; D isomer: 0.3 mg/kg/i.v./rabbits; L-isomer: 17 mg/kg/i.v./rabbits; D-iso isomer: 8.1 mg/kg/i.v./ rabbits.

Action: Hypnotic; L isomer not hypnotic; iso isomer not hypnotic; (Serotinin antagonistic).

Human Dose: 0.02-05 mg; 0.025-0.75 mg/p.o., i.m., or i.v.; 0.035-0.105 mg/p.o.

Psilocybin

3-[2-(Dimethylamino)ethyl]indol-4-ol-dihydrogen phosphate.

CY-39 (Sandoz), Indocybin® (Sandoz), psilocin phosphate ester, psilotsibin, teonanacatl].

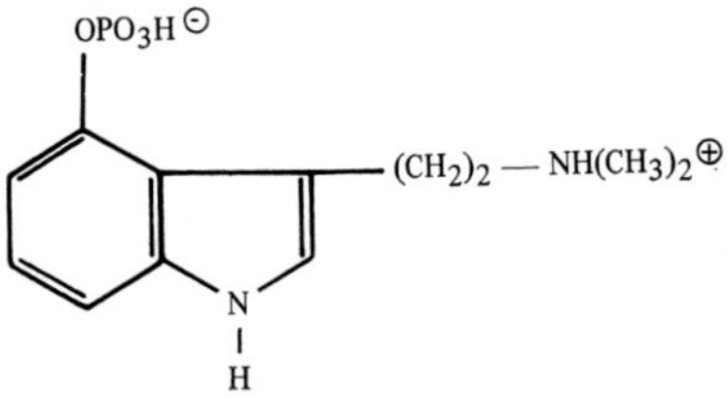
OPO3H⊖
(CH2)2 — NH(CH3)2⊕
N
H

LD_{50}: 275 mg/kg/i.v./mice; 280 mg/kg/i.v./rats; 12.5 mg/kg/i.v./rabbits.

Action: Hypnotic.

Human Dose: 4-8 mg; 6 mg/b.i.d.; 0.2 mg; 3.5-14.6 mg/p.o.; 5-14 mg/i.m.

Mescaline

3,4,5,5-Trimethoxyphenthylamine.

Mezcaline®, peyotl, TMPEA (Penick).

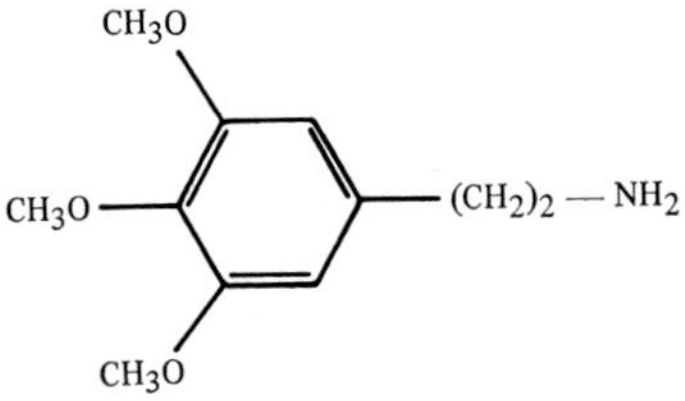
CH3O
CH3O
(CH2)2 — NH2
CH3O

LD_{50}: 500 mg/kg/i.p./mice; 157 mg/kg/i.v./mice; 534 mg/kg/i.p./mice; 370 mg/kg/i.p./rats; 157 mg/kg/i.v./rats; 534 mg/kg/s.c./rats.

Action: Hypnotic.

Human Dose: 300-600 mg; 4 mg/kg; 175-350 mg/i.m.; 490 mg/i.v.; 350 mg/p.o.

Chapter 5

ALCOHOL AND ALCOHOLISM

IT IS AN exercise in overkill to review in detail the massive chemical abuse problem that alcohol and alcoholism pose for the citizens of the United States. Estimates of alcoholics in the United States, that is, persons who are so addicted to alcohol that they have rendered themselves inadequate to meet the duties of their state in life, range from 6 million to 9 million persons. The validity of these numbers is not clear. However, there are enough alcoholics around to exert an adverse effect on every segment of our society. The problem is not one in the United States alone. It is a worldwide human problem that afflicts the communist countries as well as the noncommunist. Color is no bar to the affliction. A solution to the problem has not been discovered, nor does one seem to be in sight. Therefore, law enforcement personnel must be ready to face the results of alcohol abuse in society as it affects their job; they can be certain that the alcohol-generated emergencies of their profession will be with them for the duration of their careers.*

There is no argument about the contention that "The misuse of alcohol represents a major health problem in the United States" (Chafetz, 1972).

*Further readings in the literature of alcohol and its impact on society may be found in the following: Wilber, 1974; Seixas and Eggleston, 1976; Eckert and Noguchi, 1973; Hartroft, 1967; Saric et al., 1977; Rydberg, 1977; Blum et al., 1977; Laurell, 1977. Important and reliable information on the subject can be obtained for the asking, usually at no cost, from the National Clearinghouse for Alcohol Information, P.O. Box 2345, Rockville, Maryland 20852. In Canada, a useful and reliable quarterly publication, *Addictions,* is put out by the Alcoholism and Drug Addiction Research Foundation, 24 Harbord Street, Toronto, 5 Canada. Other valuable publications on alcohol are also available from the Foundation at modest cost.

Misinformation

The folklore surrounding alcohol and its use has caused much of the damage associated with the drug to be aggravated. For example, many drinkers believe that coffee will speed up the process of becoming sober again. Nothing is farther from the truth. Coffee may keep an individual who is under the influence of alcohol awake, but he will be a wide-awake drunk, unfit to drive or to make reliable decisions. There are other pseudoremedies for the drunk, such as breathing pure oxygen or taking a cold shower. The fact is that there is no known scientific method of speeding up the metabolism of alcohol in order to make a man return to the sober state more rapidly. As a good general rule, the average individual must allow one hour for completely getting rid of the ingested alcohol for every one-half ounce drink he imbibes. It takes as many hours to sober up as you have had drinks: two drinks, two hours to sober up; one drink, one hour to sober up.

Blood Alcohol Levels

The amount of alcohol in the blood has legal implications in the United States. In many states, a person who has 0.05 percent alcohol in the blood is *legally* concluded to be sober; he is presumed to be competent to drive an automobile under those circumstances. *Physiologically,* a person begins to show signs of impairment when the blood alcohol level reaches 0.03 to 0.05 percent.

With elevated blood alcohol content, the individual shows the following performance changes, which become greater as the blood alcohol level increases: reflex responses are slowed down, reaction time is prolonged, and complex activities such as driving an automobile, piloting a plane, or carrying out an athletic skill change for the worse. Insidiously, as these performance characteristics deteriorate, the individual believes he is performing better than without the alcohol intoxication. This distorted apprehension of reality is regularly observed in the drinking automobile driver.

Factors Influencing the Blood Alcohol Level

The rate at which alcohol gets into the blood and the resulting influence on human behavior are modified by a number of factors. One important point to remember is that alcohol is rapidly absorbed into the body from the stomach and the small intestine without any digestion; it is absorbed directly into the blood as ethanol. On the other hand, it is eliminated slowly from the body, and there is no known way of speeding up that elimination.

1. The speed of drinking influences the level of blood alcohol that results from a given volume of alcohol taken in. The more rapid the drinking, the higher will be the resulting blood alcohol level. If the drink is sipped or "nursed," the peak blood alcohol that will result is lower than if the same size drink is gulped.

2. Body weight of the drinker in terms of muscle mass is a factor; the greater the muscle mass of the body, the lower is an individual's blood alcohol level for a given amount of alcohol intake. This relationship does not include body fat; obesity, with decreased muscle mass, is no protection against alcohol. As an example, the blood alcohol level that results from the intake of 4 ounces of whiskey by a 180 pound man is significantly lower than the level reached by a 130 pound man drinking the same amount of alcohol in the same time. The bigger man, in muscle mass not fat, shows less effect of the given amount of alcohol.

3. The presence of food in the stomach retards the rate at which alcohol is absorbed. If alcohol is drunk with a large meal, the peak blood alcohol level that actually develops may be reduced by 50 percent from the theoretically maximum level.

4. Individual characteristics play a role. Under certain conditions of stress, anger, fear, or nausea, the stomach empties itself more rapidly than normal (the dumping syndrome). Under these conditions, the ingested alcohol is absorbed faster. Moreover, "a person with exten-

sive drinking problems is likely to require far more alcohol to get 'high' than an inexperienced drinker. (In individuals with serious drinking problems, the curve of tolerance is reversed, and again they are very responsive to relatively small amounts of alcohol)" (National Institute of Mental Health, 1972).

5. The type of beverage drunk does not change the active ingredient, which is ethyl alcohol. It is a natural chemical produced by a process of fermentation of sugar by the action of yeast. The concentration of alcohol in various kinds of beverages is not the same (Table 5-I). Beers, wines, and distilled spirits vary in the rate at which the alcohol they contain is absorbed by the body. The higher the concentration of alcohol in a given beverage, the faster the alcohol is absorbed. Generally, beer and wine affect a drinker more slowly than does the same amount of alcohol drunk as a distilled liquor.

Table 5-I

AMOUNTS OF ALCOHOL IN SELECTED BEVERAGES USED IN THE UNITED STATES*

Beverage	Percent Alcohol	"Proof"
Beer	2-6	3-12
Wines	14 or less	28 or less
Vodka	48	80
Whiskey	43	86
Rum	45-50	80-100
Brandy	45-55	90-110
Gin	40	80
Creme de menthe	30	60
Kummel®	39-46	78-92
Drambuie®	40	80
B and B®	43	86

*(Eckert and Noguchi, 1973)

Nevertheless, all drinks that have the same amount of alcohol will, in the end, have the same effects (Table 5-II). The rapidity with which alcohol is absorbed by the body determines how fast one becomes drunk; the rapidity with which the alcohol is me-

tabolized determines how fast one becomes sober again.   The
major part of the alcohol taken into the body is metabolized by
the liver.   The sequence of changes is as follows: Alcohol→acetal-
dehyde→acetate→intermediate   compounds→carbon   dioxide   +
water.

Table 5-II

RELATIONSHIP BETWEEN BLOOD LEVELS OF ALCOHOL
AND BEHAVIOR

Amount of Alcohol	Blood Alcohol, %	Resulting Behavior
3 ounces (2 shots)	0.05	Sedation and tranquility
6 ounces	0.10	Lack of coordination
12 ounces	0.20	Obvious intoxication
15 ounces	0.30	Unconsciousness
30 ounces	0.50 or more	Death may result

* Amount of alcohol to produce the indicated blood levels in a 155 pound
human male imbibing 90 proof whiskey on an empty stomach is shown (National Institute of Mental Health, 1972).

For every gram (0.353 fluid ounce) of alcohol metabolized by
the body, 7 calories of energy are released. Not all the alcohol in
the body is metabolized in the liver. Between 2 and 5 percent of
the total in the body is excreted *as alcohol* in the urine, breath,
and sweat.

Hangover

Hangover is an unpleasant result of the immoderate use of
alcohol. It is virtually never dangerous. The biological mechanism of hangover production is unknown. There is no medically
specific treatment for hangover, though aspirin, bed rest, and
solid food seem to alleviate the distress. Prevention consists of
nursing one's drinks, having food in the stomach, and exerting
self-discipline to avoid frank intoxication.

Biological Damage to the Body

Alcohol is a poison and should be so viewed. Quite small
amounts of alcohol taken infrequently have no known adverse
effect on the body. Large amounts taken over a prolonged period

cause chronic poisoning, including the destruction of important organs in the body.

Heart

The heart, brain, and liver seem to be the primary target organs for the toxic action of alcohol.

The muscle of the heart (myocardium) is directly harmed by large alcohol intake. The damage to the heart from alcohol is produced in the absence of known damage to any other organ such as the liver; in other words, alcohol exerts a direct poisoning action on the heart, causing a variety of heart diseases. Alcohol is so poisonous to the heart that excessive intake of the drug has brought on fatal cardiac arrest (sudden stoppage of the beat of the heart).

Digestive Tract

Stomach and duodenal ulcers are found quite often in heavy imbibers of alcohol. Alcoholic individuals also show a high incidence of chronic inflammation of the pancreas. The role of excessive alcohol intake (especially in combination with heavy cigarette smoking) is now being revealed as a demonstrable cause of cancer in the upper respiratory tract and upper portions of the alimentary tract.

Cirrhosis of the liver is more common (by factor of about 6) among alcoholics than among nonalcoholics. The mechanism of cirrhosis production by excessive alcohol intake is unknown.

Brain

Heavy intake of alcohol for many years results in grave mental disorders or permanent irreversible degeneration of the brain or peripheral nervous system. Mental functions such as memory, judgment, and learning ability can be severely damaged. Often the individual's personality structure and orientation to the real world about him break down.

The serious damage to the brain in alcoholic persons may result in a peculiar psychotic condition called *Korsakoff's syndrome*. In this condition, the victim cannot remember recent happenings.

To compensate for the defect they seem to recognize in themselves, they resort to confabulation. That is, they make up, out of whole cloth, supposed events and happenings to fill in the missing parts of the recent past. Such unfortunates seem to be in many instances victims of polyneuritis also, with burning and itching sensations in the hands and feet resulting from inflammation of the peripheral nerves. Generally these nervous system defects are not reversible. Treatment of the polyneuritis and the loss of memory with vitamins has been tried with indifferent success.

Some Statistical Information

Abusers of the drug alcohol (alcoholics) have a life expectancy of ten to twelve years less than the general public. The mortality rate for alcoholics is at least 2.5 times that of nonalcoholics. Alcoholics are also involved in a disproportionate number of violent deaths. Alcoholism is recorded on at least 13,000 death certificates each year; this number is probably grossly below the actual, for many physicians put some other cause of death on the death certificate to save the survivors embarrassment.

As a generalization, it is reasonable to make the conclusion that one-half the highway traffic fatalities are caused by alcohol. This means that about 30,000 highway fatalities per year might be eliminated or modified if chronic drinking problems could be controlled. But "public attitudes have been called the greatest single obstacle to a successful attack on the problem" (National Institute of Mental Health, 1972) .

Law enforcement personnel and prosecutors should realize that what studies have been made reveal that unless a jury is composed entirely of teetotalers, the drinkers (not necessarily abusers) invariably sympathize with the accused and "go easy" on him, perhaps motivated by the thought, "There but for the grace of God go I."

Half of homicides and about 25 percent of suicides are alcohol related. These are low estimates, but even so, almost 12,000 persons per year are represented by the percentages.

Alcohol is also involved in less violent crimes. Nearly one-half of the millions of arrests made each year in the United States are in some manner related to alcohol abuse. The number of such arrests may have declined somewhat because a few states have legislated out of existence drunkenness as a cause for arrest. Intoxicated drivers alone account for approximately 340,000 arrests in the United States each year.

The cost of the overall damage to our society resulting from the abuse of alcohol and its poisonous action on man cannot be estimated with any degree of precision other than to contend that hundreds of millions of dollars are involved and the price tag is rising with each passing year.

Drinking Drivers

Schmidt and colleagues (1973) concluded from the Katz Adjustment Scale data that male drivers involved in fatal accidents are characterized by greater shares of outgoing social aggressiveness, negativism, and psychopathology than found among males in general. They studied traffic fatalities in Baltimore, Maryland, from April 1969 to May 1972 by reviewing postmortem and toxicological analyses, General Motors collision performance and injury reports, results of mechanical dissection of vehicles, and individual motor vehicle traffic records. At autopsy, 78 percent of drivers were found to have measurable levels of blood alcohol; 52 percent had levels above .10, indicating impaired driving ability. The authors believed it reasonable to expect success in identifying high-risk drivers through multiple variable profiles and suggested the installation of passive restraining devices as a means of eliminating drivers' disregard of safety equipment. The latter recommendation is not supported by the research reported and represents a gratuitous opinion of the authors, one for which there are a number of valid objections (Schmidt et al., 1973).

According to the National Institute on Alcohol Abuse and Alcoholism (1971), the drug ethanol (ethyl alcohol, grain alcohol) can hardly be considered a safe chemical to have around the house.

Is Drinking Alcoholic Beverages Dangerous?

All substances that exert an effect on the brain have the potential to be dangerous. This is true of alcohol. Irresponsible use of alcohol includes the *heavy* risk of harming oneself or others.

On the other hand, responsible use of alcoholic beverages has been widely practiced throughout history without negative effects or consequences. Of those persons in our society who choose to drink, most do so without harm to themselves or others. Whether alcohol usage is responsible or irresponsible, harmless or danger- ous, depends of course on many factors such as the time, the place, the quantity, the reason, and the person.

For instance, alcohol starts to be a factor in automobile crashes at blood alcohol concentrations beginning as low as .05%, the approximate level reached in the average 160 pound person by consuming three 1 ounce drinks of 86 proof whiskey in an hour within two hours of eating an average meal. With little or no food in the stomach, the .05 blood alcohol concentration would be reached after approximately two drinks or two 12 ounce cans of beer consumed in an hour.

For the average healthy person, a certain amount of alcohol can be used without any lasting effects on the body or brain, but continuous drinking of large quantities can cause structural dam- age. Cirrhosis of the liver is closely linked to heavy continuous consumption of alcohol, and there is a positive correlation be- tween this type of alcohol consumption and ulcers, heart disease, and diabetes. Heavy drinking over many years may be compli- cated by serious nervous or mental disorders or may cause perma- nent brain damage. Alcohol, like many other drugs that affect the central system, can also be physiologically addicting, that is, it produces withdrawal symptoms when alcohol intake ceases.

*Even Moderate Drinking May Impair Vision**

Recent investigations have shown that even moderate doses of alcohol may possibly adversely affect vision in such a way as to impair driving ability. Research at the University of California and at the Pacific Medical Center in San Francisco, indicates that drinking, even in moderation, causes temporary but important changes in recovery from glare, identifying and visually tracking moving objects, and distinguishing between some color hues.

---

*Courtesy of National Clearinghouse for Alcohol Information, Rockville, Maryland.

The glare recovery process, even without drinking, can take many seconds or even minutes when the new light level is considerably lower than the previous level. During this time, the eye remains relatively blind to fine detail. Following alcohol ingestion, these changes in vision may last 30 to 50 percent longer. As little as one cocktail on an empty stomach in test subjects significantly prolonged recovery times following bright light exposure.

These findings, taking into account that drivers at night may be intermittently exposed to bright lights from oncoming cars and high glare from light scattered on the windshield, may help to explain why alcohol, even at low blood levels, is frequently associated with traffic accidents.

Nine men, aged twenty to twenty-eight, participated in a double-blind experiment in which two levels of alcohol dosage and a placebo were used. Following preadaptation, subjects were exposed for 10 seconds to a high-intensity light field on which a test spot was presented to gauge visual recovery. Once subjects detected the target, they operated a switch to reduce contrast a step further. Subjects were tested before drinking and at 30, 90, 180, 270, and 360 minutes after drinking, with blood alcohol levels and subjective "highs" recorded by a second experimenter at each session.

Glare recovery from a 10 second exposure to a uniform bright field was significantly retarded after alcohol ingestion. Recovery times were delayed 20 to 50 percent, depending on the quantity of alcohol taken. Predrink glare recovery values were not resumed until 6 hours after drinking.

Alcohol-induced increases in glare recovery times are dose related, this relationship is clearly evident 90 minutes after drinking, and it exists for at least 3 hours following drinking low doses of alcohol.

Alcohol ingestion had a greater effect on the visual acuity of subjects when targets were in motion. With static visual targets, there was no decrement in recognition times by subjects using socially typical doses of alcohol. However, when the targets were in motion, even one low-level dose of alcohol increased by up to 20 percent the size of object required for correct identification.

Alcohol Use and Narcotics Addiction

Alcohol plays a significant part in the scenario of drug abuse, especially of narcotics addiction (Jackson and Richman, 1973). Some workers in the field of drug abuse feel that broken down psychosocial surroundings are associated with both alcohol and narcotics abuse. The existence of a cause-and-effect relationship has not been demonstrated. Surroundings of economic deprivation are claimed to be the haven of narcotics pushers and alcohol pushers. Again the cause-and-effect relationship is dim. Whether the economic conditions bring about the addiction or whether addiction favors the drifting of the addict into such an environment is not clear. A case can be made for either alternative. Not infrequently, alcohol is used in place of heroin if the latter becomes unavailable. "Alcohol use is a major component in the natural history of narcotic addiction, the disruption of its treatment and the excess mortality suffered by the addict" (Jackson and Richman, 1973). There is strong evidence that the use of alcohol on a daily basis by heroin addicts increases the duration of the narcotic addiction. (Table 5-III).

Table 5-III
DAILY ALCOHOL USE AS RELATED TO LENGTH OF DRUG ADDICTION
AND OTHER STATISTICS*

Statistic	*Years of Addiction*			
	0-2	*3-5*	*6-15*	*16+*
Total sample (%)	7%	23%	33%	46%
Sex				
Male	5	27	32	43
Female	10	12	39	71
Age				
25	10	22	23	—
25-34	0	25	30	40
35	—	—	29	50
Ethnicity				
Hispanic	4	19	22	39
Non-Hispanic black	5	26	43	51
Non-Hispanic white	17	17	27	—
First admission	8	25	29	28
Readmission	—	20	36	53
Heroin alone	0	12	13	38
Heroin and other drugs	25	41	47	55

*(Jackson and Richman, 1973)

In one study, it was found that almost one-half of the heroin addicts in the population investigated used a number of other drugs on a daily basis. Alcohol was used by about 13 percent of addicts using only heroin. Addicts using other drugs besides heroin showed a 44 percent frequency of regular alcohol use. More than 40 percent of the polydrug users (barbiturates, cocaine, methadone, or glutethimide plus heroin) also were found to use alcohol on a daily basis.

The impression among some experts in the field of drug abuse that in recent years there has been an increased "lethality" of narcotic addiction may stem from the greater frequency (which continues to grow) of polydrug abuse, including the damaging action of alcohol.

Alcohol or Carbon Monoxide?

The question has been posed a number of times whether carbon monoxide may in fact be the lethal agent in some of the 30,000 or more deaths each year on our nation's highway's now attributed to the poisonous effects of ethanol on drivers. Alcohol has been shown to be far more significant than carbon monoxide *and other drugs* (alcohol obviously is a drug) in fatal automobile accidents (Davis, 1974). This conclusion is based on a study made of fatal automobile accidents in Dade County, Florida, over a period of twelve years. Routine toxicological investigations by the medical examiner of Dade County revealed that alcohol was the intoxicant (poisoning agent) most frequently involved in driver fatalities in the twelve-year period. Carbon monoxide as a major cause of fatal accidents was insignificant compared with alcohol. Drugs other than alcohol were found upon occasion. Evidence of chemicals other than alcohol or carbon monoxide was found in 5.6 percent of drivers killed immediately in road accidents and in 9 percent of those drivers killed in single-vehicle accidents.

It is obvious that attempts to explain away alcohol as *the* lethal agent in highway automobile deaths is futile. Moreover, a significant number of driver deaths from road accidents may reveal no alcohol or carbon monoxide of note in the blood of the deceased, but in nearly 6 percent of these cases other drugs may be demonstrable. The 9 percent of dead drivers involved in one-car accidents who show no blood alcohol nor carbon monoxide but do reveal other drugs in the blood pose a serious question about all so-called unexplainable one-car accidents. It is safe to hypothesize that if dead drivers from these one-car accidents were all subjected to thorough toxicological workup, the vast majority would be shown to have blood alcohol levels that impaired their driving; most of the balance would have other drugs in their blood at levels that could bring about a performance decrement. An insignificant number would have lethal levels of carbon monoxide in the blood. Virtually none of these cases would be truly "unexplained." Under present conditions of limited legal demands for complete toxicological workup of drivers killed on the highway and in the face of chronic budget limitations for medical examiners or coroners (especially the latter) to carry out their assigned duties, it may be many years before this hypothesis can be put to the test. It does seem appropriate to urge that the influence on the number of driver deaths from carbon monoxide and drugs other than alcohol and from combinations of intoxicants be studied with increased intensity in keeping with the fiscal realities of our various medicolegal systems.

Plane Crashes

Civilian aviation accidents are clearly related to what is properly called *abuse of alcohol*. Lacefield (1975) has reported a consistent increase in these accidents by an overall factor of more than 4 times in a period of about six years. In 1974, 9 percent of the civilian pilots killed in crashes had blood alcohol levels of over 50 mg/100 ml of blood at the time of the crash. Alcohol was found in 359 pilots involved in 44 percent of airplane crashes studied by Lacefield and covering a seven-year span of time. Other contributing factors to these crash deaths include drugs, carbon monoxide levels at dangerous values, and cyanide in the blood (derived from burning cabin materials). Nevertheless, the contribution of these latter materials was comparatively unimportant in the overall picture; alcohol clearly is shown to play the major role in civilian plane crashes.

These facts suggest that two endeavors seem warranted in the future. First of all, there must be launched a much more vigorous and effective indoctrination program for civilian pilots concerning the serious dangers associated with drinking and piloting. Secondly, every effort should be made to require a reasonably complete toxicological workup of all pilots involved in fatal crashes in order to arrive at a clearer more comprehensive understanding of the chemical hazards posed for the civilian pilot.

In Great Britain, the pattern is much the same with respect to the role of excessive alcohol in the fatal failures of civilian pilots. The following all too typical case illustrates the point (Underwood Ground, 1975).

> Impairment of flying skills by alcohol was identified as the principal factor leading to the death of an experienced pilot and two passengers in the crash landing of a three-seat light cabin monoplane. The liver of the pilot showed diffuse fatty changes, and toxicological examination revealed alcohol in concentrations of 149 mg/100 ml in the blood and 139 mg/100 ml in the urine. On initial screening for drugs, the presence of nitrazepam and chlordiazepoxide was suspected, and the medical investigation was complicated by the finding of chlordiazepoxide in the personal effects. Although the cause of the accident was listed as a low-altitude stall during an attempted forced landing following loss of engine power, it was concluded that alcohol had adversely affected the pilot's ability to avoid onset of the stall.

Should BAC Samples be Refrigerated?

The ethanol concentration in a contaminated specimen of postmortem blood was measured under different temperature conditions, and the effect of fluoride on microbial production of ethanol was determined. Ethanol concentration increased from 5 to 18 mg/dl (deciliter) upon storage of the specimen for several hours at room temperature. The concentration increased to 44 mg/dl after a day's refrigeration, and to 87 mg/dl after an additional period of incubation at 35°C. Five microorganisms were isolated from the specimen, and all were shown capable of producing ethanol when cultured in bank blood. Of these organisms, *Proteus vulgaris* and alpha-streptococci produced relatively little ethanol, and this production was eliminated or reduced to undetectable levels by fluoride. However, *Candida albicans* produced a much greater amount of ethanol, and this production was not at all inhibited by fluoride (Blume and Lakatua, 1973) . Therefore, it is recommended that blood samples for alcohol analysis have sodium fluoride added and that the drawn samples be cooled quickly and be refrigerated until the analysis for alcohol is begun.

Blood alcohol levels at various intervals after alcohol ingestion and after drinker involvement in an accident were evaluated and correlated to rates of alcohol elimination. The blood alcohol level within 2 hours after an incident may be considered to be not significantly different from the level at the time of the incident because the rate of change during this time is less than the analytical error of the test procedure (Loomis, 1974) . This information is important to the law enforcement officer in the event a defense attorney argues any delay in taking a blood alcohol test as cause for throwing out the results as evidence. On the other hand, investigating officers should insure that blood alcohol tests are made within 2 hours of an accident because the results will then be essentially identical with the values that prevailed at the time of the incident.

A Blood Alcohol Formula

Zink and Reinhardt (1976) have generated a prediction equation for calculating the blood alcohol level in a person at the time a specified event occurred derived from the blood alcohol level ascertained at the time the sample was taken. The equation is based on over 2000 individual cases in which serial samples of blood have been analyzed for alcohol content. The computer-generated prediction equation follows:

Maximal alcohol concentration (gm%) = concentration in sample (gm%) + 0.02 (gm%) + 0.02 (gm%) per hour.

According to the authors, the equation predicts with a confidence level of 99 percent. They conclude that, "The formula is valid for all common forms of drinking in the rising and falling parts of blood alcohol curvature."

Breath Alcohol

There is now general agreement that measurement of breath alcohol levels cannot replace blood alcohol levels in cases of forensic interest *(Citation,* 1973; German commisson, 1976; Mason and Dubowski, 1976). Although Mason and Dubowski propose a statutory definition of the offense *driving under the influence of alcohol* to be based on the amount of ethanol in the breath, there are methodological considerations that call such a definition into question. One of the chief weaknesses of breath alcohol estimation is that full cooperation of the subject is needed in following instructions for exhaling. The opportunity for the shrewd subject to breathe in such a manner as to give low breath alcohol levels exists; it will always render breath alcohol measurements suspect.

There is no reason that breath alcohol measurements cannot be used to establish "probable cause" (much like the roadside tests are used) for demanding a blood alcohol test.

Blood and Urine Alcohol

If blood or urine be measured for alcohol content, the result

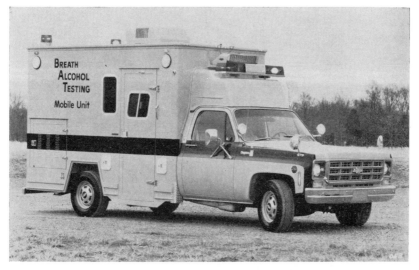

Figure 5-1. A mobile breath alcohol testing unit houses a breath alcohol measuring system and can be so constructed as to provide facilities for booking and holding subjects and storage of data and supplies. The illustrated commercial unit is referred to as the FACT BATmobile. Courtesy of First Ambulance Center of Tennessee, Inc. (FACT), Shelbyville, Tennessee.

provides a basis for concluding how much beer or whiskey was consumed (Tables 5-IV and 5-V).

Table 5-IV
BEER CONSUMPTION, BASED ON ALCOHOL CONTENT

Blood Alcohol mg/100 ml	Urine Alcohol mg/100 ml	Beer Pints
18	24	0.5
37	49	1.0
73	97	2.0
147	196	4.0
201	268	5.5
366	488	10.0

Table 5-V
WHISKEY CONSUMPTION, BASED ON ALCOHOL CONTENT

Blood Alcohol mg/100 ml	Urine Alcohol mg/100 ml	Whiskey Ounces
22	30	1
45	660	2
67	90	3
135	180	6
225	300	10
360	480	16
562	750	25

The relationship between blood alcohol and urine alcohol is variable and may be influenced by many factors. For legal purposes, blood alcohol is the reference standard; urine alcohol levels (and for that matter, breath alcohol levels) are indicative much as clinical examinations by a physician may be indicative of incapacitation by alcohol. For courtroom use, the standard is the level of alcohol in the blood.

Legal Intoxication

There is growing evidence that so-called medical tests for legal or criminal intoxication may be of no scientific value (Solarz, 1975). A study of 646 cases in which the urine alcohol was 0.4 gm or more per 100 ml also included the results of medical tests administered by physicians to ascertain whether the subjects were drunk or not. In only 25 percent of the cases did the physicians' observations using clinical tests agree with the degree of intoxication revealed by the respective levels of alcohol in blood and urine. Apparently overt signs and symptoms (as revealed by clinical tests) of alcohol intoxication do not necessarily match high alcohol levels in body fluids. For example, persons who have developed ethanol tolerance are predisposed to exhibiting few overt signs of drunkenness. Moreover, degree of outward intoxication may reflect other factors including nutrition, amount of sleep, or fatigue. The subjective responses of the examining physician may also modify the results; at present there is no way to standardize or make quantitative the physician's subjective view.

Autopsy results obtained from automobile accident victims having severe head injuries indicate that the alcohol content of blood clots inside the skull is significantly higher than the alcohol content of the blood taken from the heart of the same victim. In four of the cases, the victims had survived several hours from time of injury to time of death. These results suggest that the alcohol content of intracranial (inside the skull) blood clots may be a valuable index of the state of intoxication at the time of the accident (Freireich et al., 1975). It may be useful for investigating police officers to ask that the pathological examination included in a postmortem study of automobile accident victims cover analysis of intracranial blood clots for alcohol content.

The Situation in New Mexico

A review of drinking and driving in the State of New Mexico, which does not have a coroner's system but has instituted an effective state medical investigator system for handling violent, suspicious, or unattended deaths, presents in broad terms the alcohol-automobile fatality picture quite representative of that seen across the nation.

The experience with drinking and driving in New Mexico serves as a useful way to summarize one of the major effects of alcohol on individuals and on society.

About Drinking and Driving in New Mexico*

A number of studies have been conducted in several states to determine the blood alcohol content of traffic fatalities. These studies have shown that between 20 and 70% of drivers who died in traffic accidents had a significant blood alcohol (B.A.) level; i.e., greater than 0.01%. The percentages of pedestrian and passenger fatalities who had a significant B.A. were similar but somewhat lower.

We decided to look retrospectively at traffic fatalities in New Mexico and chose to include traffic fatalities which were reported to the OMI from July 1974 to June 1976. During this period there were 875 traffic fatalities in New Mexico and we divided this total group into truck and auto drivers (n = 418), truck and auto passengers (n = 246), pedestrians (n = 172), and drivers and passengers on motorcycles (n = 39). We also subdivided the total study group by age and by location (county). The blood alcohol was determined by gas chromatography using an internal standard head space method with a precision of 7% (2 S.D.).

Type of Fatality

We found that 36% of all fatalities had a significant B.A. (greater than 0.01%), 30% had a B.A. greater than the legal intoxication limit of 0.10%, and 8% had a B.A. above a stated lethal limit of 0.40%. These figures agree with those from studies in other states except for the extremely high alcohol levels. We feel that the 8% represents an unusually high percent. Although there are no other studies available for direct comparison, a recent study of acute alcohol poisoning in North Carolina shows that a significant number of persons with B.A.s greater than 0.40% died in traffic accidents.

A large portion of the total traffic fatalities were male (650 of 875 or 74%) and, of those fatalities who had significant blood alcohol levels, an even higher percentage were male (265 or 319 or 83%).

We subdivided the traffic fatalities according to whether the

*Courtesy of James T. Weston, M.D., Editor, *Newsletter,* Office of the Medical Investigator State of New Mexico, Albuquerque, New Mexico

deceased was the driver, a passenger, or a pedestrian, and the data are shown in Table 5-VI. Surprisingly, a larger percentage of fatally injured motorcyclists had significant blood alcohol levels compared to drivers of autos and trucks. Not so surprising was the higher percentage of pedestrians who had a B.A. above the legal intoxication limit of 0.10%. Additionally, the pedestrians had the highest average B.A. (0.287%) while the motorcyclists had the lowest (0.178%). The average B.A. in fatally injured drivers (0.217%) compares well with an average of 0.220% found in a large study of drivers in Dallas, Texas in 1966. Another interesting comparison is the highest B.A.s found in the various groups. The drivers had the highest extreme level (0.650%) while the motorcyclists had the lowest extreme level (0.268%).

Table 5-VI
FATAL TRAFFIC ACCIDENTS AND ALCOHOL IN NEW MEXICO
JULY 1974 TO JUNE 1976

	Percentage Pos. Alcohol (>.01%)	Percentage Legally Intox. (>.10%)	Mean Alcohol Level	Highest Alcohol Level
Pedestrians	40% 69 of 172	38% 65 of 172	.287%	.570%
Drivers	39% 164 of 418	32% 133 of 418	.217%	.650%
Passengers	28% 64 of 246	17% 43 of 246	.178%	.550%
Motorcyclists	44% 17 of 39	33% 13 of 39	.165%	.268%
TOTAL	36% 319 of 875	30% 260 of 875	.221%	.650%

Another significant comparison was obtained when we grouped the fatalities according to age (Table 5-VII). Although the data in some age groups may be distorted because of the small number of fatalities, some general statements can be made:

1. 50% of the fatalities were between 16 and 30 years old.
2. The percentage of males with significant alcohol is generally high for all fatalities between 20 and 60 years old, while the percentage of females with significant alcohol continues to rise with age and is highest for

Table 5-VII

TRAFFIC FATALITIES IN NEW MEXICO (1974-76)
AGE AND SEX VS. BLOOD ALCOHOL

Age	0-10	11-15	16-20	21-25	26-30	31-35	36-40	41-45	46-50	51-55	56-60	61-65	66-70	71-75
Males														
1. Number of traffic deaths	25	12	90	101	50	41	24	25	16	30	15	18	17	10
2. % of total	4.0	2.0	14.8	16.5	8.1	6.7	3.9	4.1	2.6	4.9	2.5	3.0	2.9	1.6
3. % with alcohol	0	25.	44.	57.	38.	46.	33.	40.	62.	37.	27.	28.	24.	10.
4. Average B.A.	—	.098	.152	.218	.270	.288	.239	.236	.220	.322	.328	.273	.355	.238
Females														
1. Number of traffic deaths	13	8	29	18	14	9	14	8	13	3	5	11	7	10
2. % of total	2.1	1.3	4.7	3.0	2.4	1.5	2.4	.13	2.2	<1	<1	1.8	1.1	1.6
3. % with alcohol	0	25.	27.	17.	21.	33.	36.	50.	38.	33.	0	9.	0	10.
4. Average B.A.	—	.277	.144	.244	.342	.337	.271	.338	.347	.158	—	.272	0	.022

fatalities between 40 and 50 years old.

3. The average blood alcohol for both males and females is higher with age; however the average for females is highest between 30 and 50 years.

The study illustrates several facets of alcohol-related traffic fatalities in New Mexico. For instance, more than one-third of all such fatalities had significant alcohol. While a large percentage of these fatalities (30%) were males between 15 and 30 years old, higher average blood alcohols generally were found in females and older males. A higher percentage of pedestrian fatalities were legally intoxicated, but blood alcohol was detected in a higher percentage of motorcyclists.

The results of the study of drinking and driving in New Mexico are in accord with findings from other studies made on the problem. In the New Mexico data, only fatally injured persons are included. Cross-comparison with studies that include nonfatal traffic incidents must be made with extreme caution. There is inadequate information about survivors of accidents in this study and in others. No quantitative information here or in other studies published in the usually available scientific literature is obtainable to answer the popular claim that a drunk involved in an accident comes off better than a sober person because the drunk is relaxed all over and behaves like a rag doll when involved in a crash. Intuitively one is led to discard the claim; data would be helpful.

General Conclusion

Alcohol must be considered a toxic drug that is more widely abused than any other chemical. Its damage to individuals and to society from abuse exceeds that resulting from all other abused drugs added together.

The pathology caused by alcohol in abusing individuals encompasses every organ system in the body (National Clearinghouse for Alcohol Information, 1976).

As a poisonous chemical posing clear and present danger to human beings, alcohol must be given first place.

Chapter 6

TOXIC GASES

TOXIC OR noxious gases may be classified from the point of view of respiration as follows.

IRRITANTS. These injure the air passages and produce inflammation of the respiratory tract.

ASPHYXIANTS. *Simple asphyxiants* are chemically inert, for example, hydrogen or nitrogen; they act mechanically to smother a victim. Most heating gases are simple asphyxiants except for some that, in limited parts of the United States, contain carbon monoxide. *Chemical asphyxiants* are exemplified by carbon monoxide, which combines with the hemoglobin in the blood and renders it inactive for transporting oxygen. Others in this group act on some cellular constituent to prevent tissues from using the oxygen that may be delivered to them.

VOLATILE DRUGS. These inhalants have no direct effect on the lungs. They act only after absorption into the bloodstream and transport to the tissues of the body. They seem to act at the surface of cells. The anesthetic gases and the volatile hydrocarbons of industry are examples.

INORGANIC AND ORGANOMETALLIC SUBSTANCES.

In general, the treatment for any of these toxic inhalants is the same: (1) rapid elimination of poison through the lungs, the site of entry; (2) oxygen therapy; and (3) antidote for poison that acts systemically.

Some physiological characteristics of various noxious gases are shown in Table 6-I.

Table 6-I
SOME PHYSIOLOGICAL CHARACTERISTICS OF VARIOUS NOXIOUS
GASES*

Gas	Maximum Allowable Concentration Over 1 hour	½ to 1 hour	Throat Irritation Short Exposure
Hydrogen chloride	10	50-100	35
Ammonia	85-100	300-500	408
Hydrogen fluoride	3	10	—
Formaldehyde	20	—	—
Sulfur dioxide	10	50-100	8-12
Chlorine	0.35-1.0	4	15
Phosphorus trichloride	0.1 -0.15	4	—
Bromine	<0.7	<2-4	—
Nitrous oxides	10-40	100-150	62
Phosgene	1.0 or less	25	3.1
Arsine	1	6-30	—
Hydrogen sulfide	20	170-300	—

*Values are given in parts per million of toxicant in the inspired air.

The Unit of Measurement

If the concentration of a gas is given as *parts per million* (ppm), it is meant that so many parts of a chemical (carbon monoxide or nitrogen oxide, for example) as a vapor are mixed with 1 million parts of air *by volume:* volumes of gas/million volumes of air. The unit is confused however.

In contrast, some toxicologists use *parts per million* to mean parts of a distinct chemical in 1 million parts of the total air-contaminant mixture. As an illustration, 1 ppm SO_2 in air means (in this definition) that one volume of SO_2 had enough air added to it to bring the total volume up to 1 million volume units (1 ml SO_2 + 999,999 ml air).

In low concentrations, the difference between the two is trivial; at high levels of contamination of air, the difference may be significant.

If the contaminant is solid (dust or aerosol), the usual expression is 1 milligram (mass) of particle per 1 million parts of air (by volume); the conventional way of expressing this value is milligrams of contaminant per cubic meter of air.

CARBON MONOXIDE*
Some Chemical Facts

Carbon monoxide is a gas that is poisonous to human beings. It has no odor nor taste; it is colorless. Only rarely is it found free in nature in any but small amounts. Tobacco smoke contains significantly large amounts of carbon monoxide: Smoke from cigarettes has 1 percent by volume of carbon monoxide; pipe smoke, 2 percent; cigar smoke, 6 percent. These amounts present clear hazards to human health (Dominquez, 1962; Finck, 1966).

The gas dissolves only slightly in water; at $0°C$, one volume of water dissolves about 0.04 volume of carbon monoxide; at $20°C$, about 0.02 volume.

Internal combustion engines produce large amounts of carbon monoxide. It has been said that automobile exhaust contains about 3 pounds of carbon monoxide for every gallon of gasoline burned (Spitz and Fisher, 1973). Although carbon monoxide will not support combustion, it burns (is combustible) in the presence of air with a blue flame, forming carbon dioxide.

Protection

Special respirators (gas masks) are available with canisters that contain *hopcalite*. Carbon monoxide passes through such a canister and is oxidized (burned) at room temperature to form harmless carbon dioxide. Hopcalite is a chemical mixture made up as follows:

> Manganese dioxide, 50 percent
> Copper oxide, 30 percent
> Cobaltic oxide, 15 percent
> Silver oxide, 5 percent

Heat is given off in large amounts during the process of converting the carbon monoxide to carbon dioxide; hence the canisters quick-

---

*"Carbon monoxide is by far the most important single cause of strictly accidental poisoning. It may be formed by incomplete combustion of any carbonaceous material, including natural gas. However, natural gas, unlike manufactured fuel gases, does not contain preformed carbon monoxide, and, therefore simple leaks of natural gas offer far less toxic hazard. Carbon monoxide ranks second only to alcohol as a direct cause of fatal intoxication" (Hayes, 1975).

ly become hot during use. These canisters do *not* protect against any other toxic gas.

Identification of Carbon Monoxide

There are commercially available tubes enclosing special chemicals that change color in the presence of carbon monoxide; the intensity of the color varies directly with the amount of carbon monoxide present (Fig. 6-1). Automated continuously recording devices, some with alarms that go off at the danger point for carbon monoxide in air, are also commercially available. Digital readout meters are also available (Figs. 6-2 and 6-3). Other companies sell similar devices (Figs. 6-4 and 6-5).

Most biochemical laboratories and major hospital clinical laboratories are equipped to perform carbon monoxide tests on samples of air and of blood. For example, Carle Instruments Inc. has apparatus that can measure even minute traces of carbon monoxide in air using a gas chromatograph procedure. Essentially, carbon monoxide is catalytically changed to methane in this method after necessary separation by gas chromatography. The instrument then uses a sensitive flame-ionization detector to calibrate carbon monoxide in air in ppm. The detection limit is .05 ppm. The system can be automated.

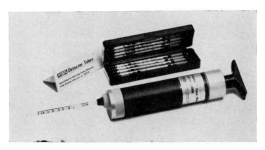

Figure 6-1. A hand pump model of indicator of carbon monoxide in air. A calibrated glass tube is inserted into a special hand pump. The tube contains a special chemical reagent that changes to a specified color when carbon monoxide comes in contact with it. Spread of the color along the length of the tube indicates the amount of carbon monoxide in the sample of air drawn through it. Courtesy of Mine Safety Appliances Company, Pittsburg, Pennsylvania.

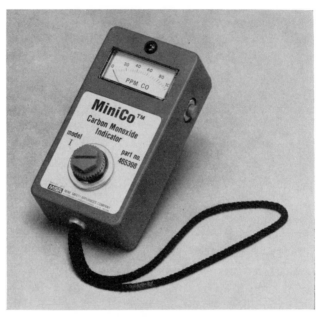

Figure 6-2. A hand-carried miniature carbon monoxide indicator has a digital readout, giving parts per million of carbon monoxide directly on the readout face. Courtesy of Mine Safety Appliances Company, Pittsburgh, Pennsylvania.

Man's Role in Producing Carbon Monoxide

"As the industrial revolution advances and spreads, more carbon monoxide than formerly becomes produced through the incomplete combustion of carbon compounds" (Allen and Allard, 1961).

Claude Bernard, the renowned French physiologist of the nineteenth century (he is held to be the father of modern physiology), first demonstrated clearly that carbon monoxide has a much greater affinity for hemoglobin (the red coloring matter in the human blood) than does oxygen by a factor of several hundred.

The history of the hazard posed by carbon monoxide to man is long and impressive. Automobiles produce large amounts of carbon monoxide and thus become tools of accidental, homicidal, and suicidal deaths. Moreover, it is now apparent that in the latter

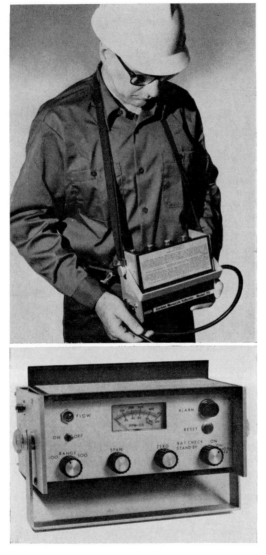

Figure 6-3. A portable carbon monoxide indicator with a range wide enough to satisfy most needs. A probe can be introduced into any area or container to pick up air sample to be tested for carbon monoxide. An alarm can be set to go off at any level deemed dangerous for a specific purpose. Courtesy of Mine Safety Appliances Company, Pittsburgh, Pennsylvania.

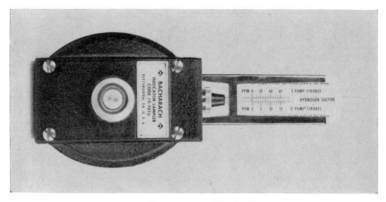

Figure 6-4. MONOXOR® carbon monoxide indicator. The concentration of carbon monoxide is shown by the length of the stain in the indicator tube and measured on the etched scale of the instrument. No color comparison is required. CO concentrations as low as 0.005% can be measured. Courtesy of Bacharach Instrument Company, Pittsburg, Pennsylvania.

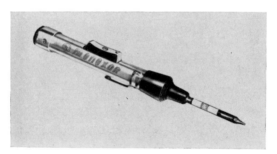

Figure 6-5. MONOXOR® carbon monoxide detector is intended to detect dangerous carbon monoxide concentrations. CO concentrations as low as 100 ppm of air can be revealed instantly. Courtesy of Bacharach Instrument Company, Pittsburgh, Pennsylvania.

part of the twentieth century, carbon monoxide generated by automobiles has become a significant manmade environmental threat to mankind. Cities like Denver and Los Angeles have periodic alerts during which the ill and the elderly are cautioned to stay indoors and reduce their physical activity to a minimum in the face of hazardous levels of carbon monoxide as an air pollutant. The concentration of carbon monoxide in the atmosphere of urban areas in the United States has been reported at 1 to 200 ppm (Loomis, 1968).

The combination of carbon monoxide with hemoglobin of the blood results in the production of carboxyhemoglobin (Wilber, 1966). The reaction is reversible:

$$HbO_2 + CO \rightleftharpoons HbCO + O_2$$

Carbon Monoxide Source*

Most investigators are familiar with automobile exhaust fumes as one of the principal sources of carbon monoxide. We emphasize the importance of automobile exhaust with the engine running only a relatively short time within a closed space and the large volume of carbon monoxide that may be generated from such a source. We also emphasize the relatively small amount of carbon monoxide that it takes to bind the oxygen-carrying hemoglobin contained within the erythrocytes (red blood cells) of the blood so that they no longer are capable of carying oxygen from the lungs to the vital structures of the body, thereby causing death as a result of *chemical asphyxia*. We concur with the importance of on-scene investigation of deaths that occur in garages as well as deaths that occur in parked automobiles, whether or not the engine is running at the time the individual is discovered. Often detailed examination of the motor vehicle and its exhaust system, together with examination of the interior of the automobile, to determine if carbon monoxide is transmitted therein is the only way of identifying the source of this gas. Investigators would do well to also consider carbon monoxide as a possible cause for unexplained accidents, particularly in older model automobiles.

In addition to motor vehicle exhaust, carbon monoxide is generated in any incomplete combustion, that is, in any fire in which there are not liberal amounts of oxygen present to support such combustion. This condition would include, but is not necessarily limited to, the following typical circumstances:

1. A typical house conflagration where death occurs much

*Courtesy of James T. Weston, M.D., Editor, *Newsletter,* Office of the Medical Investigator, State of New Mexico, Albuquerque, New Mexico.

more frequently from carbon monoxide than from inhalation of smoke or soot or thermal burns.

2. A poorly ventilated house heater, particularly prone to occur in the fall of the year when obstructions to the vent of the chimney or within the chimney have not been identified.

3. Inadequately ventilated heating devices. This situation might include wall furnaces wherein there are too many curves within the flue pipe or furnaces in which the maximum diameter of the flue is not in keeping with those demonstrated to be necessary in recent years, such that when the furnace runs continuously for a long period of time, the level of carbon monoxide progressively increases. This type of situation is most apt to occur in sustained periods of cold weather.

4. Incompletely burned gas within leaking hot water heaters wherein water, brought in contact with the carbon soot deposits within the flue and on the burners, serves as a catalyst to produce excessive carbon monoxide.

5. When completely unvented devices such as catalytic heaters or charcoal burners are moved from the exterior where they have ample oxygen to the interiors of campers, trailers, or even outhouses.

There is a common misconception that natural gas contains large quantities of carbon monoxide, when in fact it does not. Manufactured gas, usually prepared along the eastern and western seaboards from the burning of coal or coke, does contain large quantities of carbon monoxide and may, in and of itself, cause carbon monoxide poisoning in the event a gas jet is left open or a burner with a faulty safety device is extinguished. Natural gas may produce death, but it is usually by *mechanical suffocation,* that is, the replacement of air containing the necessary oxygen by natural gas itself.

Law enforcement officers are encouraged to impart the risk of inadequately ventilated heaters and motor vehicles in need of repair to members of families and friends within their community.

It would be well, as a public service, to advise groups within the community of the extreme risk of these devices or of transporting charcoal or other unvented or portable heaters to the interior of homes during extremes of cold.

Findings on a Carbon Monoxide Victim

The most obvious finding on a victim of carbon monoxide poisoning is the bright cherry red coloration of the skin in those places where dependent lividity is apparent. This may vary from wine color to cherry red, is usually quite splotchy, and when excessive, is usually accompanied by a blistering change in the skin, which is readily slipped from the underlying tissues. These blisters resemble those of thermal burns or of the kind of change associated with exposure to a solvent such as gasoline and are not too dissimilar from the early changes of postmortem autolysis, except that other autolytic changes associated with decomposition are not apparent. These signs may be, and usually are, the only findings apparent on the exterior of a carbon monoxide victim. It is important to remember that individuals who do not have very much blood, either by virtue of anemia or hemorrhage near the time of death, may not have readily apparent external coloration of the skin, since there is not sufficient blood to be colored for this to be visible through the surface of the skin.

There may be evidence that the victim has vomited just before his death. Other individuals present who are not deceased may be unconscious or conscious, with a tendency to vomit, and almost invariably complaining of headache. Prompt medical attention should be provided to all surviving individuals suspected to have been exposed to carbon monoxide.

Chemical Examination

A good whole blood specimen is necessary to rule out or determine the degree of carbon monoxide poisoning. If there is even the most remote suspicion that carbon monoxide may have caused death or contributed to an accident that, in turn, resulted in death, in addition to the vitreous sample, a good blood sample should be taken. This requirement may necessitate the opening of the body cavity in order to remove a sample not in contact with other body fluids and with red blood clots in addition to the serum.

When it is important to know immediately whether or not the individual expired as a result of carbon monoxide poisoning in order to prevent exposure of others to the same risk, the investigator should seek the services of a local laboratory, suggesting that they conduct a dilution test, that is, a test accomplished simply by putting one or two drops of the blood removed from the victim in a test tube of water and shaking vigorously. In carbon monoxide deaths, this usually retains a bright red color. The test should always be controlled by putting one or two drops of blood from an individual known not to be exposed to carbon monoxide in similar fluid and comparing the two. This is not a definitive or confirmatory test, but simply a screening test to be used only as a lifesaving device locally.

Usually levels of 30% to 40% saturation are necessary to consider CO to be the cause of death. In young adults, carbon monoxide levels are very often in the magnitude of 80% to 95% saturated. In older individuals with preexisting natural disease such as coronary atherosclerosis or cerebral atherosclerosis, death may occur at considerably lower levels.

When it is suspected or has been determined that an individual expired as a result of carbon monoxide poisoning, either in a vehicle or as a result of a faulty device within the home, the investigating agency should bring this to the attention of the local police department and the local agency responsible for building conditions. The law enforcement agencies should be advised that the house or vehicle is a threat to life in its present condition and should be sealed and impounded until remedial action has been taken, following which the licensing or inspecting agency should verify the correction of this condition before allowing occupation of the residence or use of the vehicle. *This simple expedient can put you in the business of saving lives during cold days.* Many people do not realize that they have a hole in their muffler and that a parked vehicle with the heater fan activated may readily draw exhaust fumes through the floor of the vehicle and render the person initially unconscious and then cause death. Particularly risky is the practice of allowing small children to sleep on the floor of closed vehicles or on the rear seat while the vehicle is parked.

Special Circumstances

Of particular concern in some areas is the possibility that low levels of carbon monoxide may cause the individual to present the appearance of intoxication or lose consciousness while driving his motor vehicle. This is more apt to occur in locations where the altitude is above that of mean sea level and the consequent concentration of carbon monoxide to which the individual is exposed is relatively greater. This is why the blood sample, in addition to the vitreous, should be obtained on all unexplained single-passenger motor vehicle accidents. Blood alcohol determination is readily accomplished on the vitreous, but the carbon monoxide determination is performed only on whole blood.

Other Conditions Producing Color Changes on the Body

There are three conditions that result in red coloration of the exterior of the body. During cold weather, by far the most common is cold itself. This coloration of the body may even occur after death if the individual is thereafter exposed to cold and frequently occurs when bodies are refrigerated. Carbon monoxide is the second most common cause of the red coloration and much more frequently encountered than the third, cyanide poisoning.

CYANIDE. Cyanide poisoning produces a red coloration of the body because the cyanide prevents the erythrocytes (red blood cells) from releasing the oxygen they normally carry from the lungs to the tissues, thereby presenting the appearance of arterial blood rather than the blue coloration of venous blood. If cyanide poisoning is suspected, a detailed postmortem examination should be done. Appropriate toxicology samples should be collected. Often the only additional but inconsistent clue to the presence of cyanide, a relatively unusual finding, is the characteristic odor of almonds emanating usually from the gastric contents.

Other coloration apparent on the exterior of the body that

might be encountered is the blue color, commonly referred to as cyanosis, which in some of the older textbooks is described as occurring in a number of conditions. It might be generally stated that in any location in which blood comes close enough to the surface to be apparent, this blood almost invariably turns blue if it remains there after death, so *there is virtually no significance to the presence of cyanosis or blue coloration on a deceased person, whether it be on the fingernail beds, lips, toenails or mucus membranes of the mouth.*

METHEMOGLOBINEMIA. Another unusual external coloration that might be encountered considerably less frequently is the brown bronzing of the skin, mucous membranes, and blood vessels of the eyes incident to methemoglobinemia. This condition, wherein the hemoglobin within the erythrocytes is combined into a brown-colored complex, is the condition that was first described after exposure to nitrites and nitrates and that resulted in change of the chemical composition of the wax crayons presently available for children to play with. This same brown coloration may occur as the result of nitrite contamination in a number of water supplies. Methemoglobineima, resulting again in decreased oxygen-carrying capacity of the blood, does not usually occur in adults since the enzyme system necessary to convert this is sufficiently active that it prevents excessive accumulation of this complex. This is not true in infants and very young children, in whom the enzyme has not progressed to the point where this complex is destroyed as fast as it is formed.

JAUNDICE. One final coloration most experienced investigators have probably already encountered is that associated with the accumulation of bile pigments within the blood, namely, jaundice or the yellow-green coloration particularly apparent in the sclera or white of the eye in its earliest stages, but readily apparent over all of the surface of the skin as it progresses.

Automobile Air Conditioners

It is fairly widely known that sitting in a closed car during cold weather with the engine running and the heater operating is courting death by carbon monoxide poisoning. Not so widely appreciated is the danger of sitting in a closed car on a hot day with the engine running and the air conditioner operating. Death can result. For example, in mid-July 1978 during a humid, hot spell in Queens, New York, a thirteen-year-old female and a nineteen-year-old male were found dead in a parked car. They had been chatting with the windows closed, the engine running, and the air conditioner operating. Carbon monoxide killed them (*New York Times*, 1978).

Carboxyhemoglobin

This compound is made up of four molecules of carbon monoxide attached to four iron atoms in the hemoglobin. Hemoglobin itself consists of four molecules of heme combined with globin. The iron exists in the ferrous state; it has two bonds for entering into chemical combinations. The iron in hemoglobin is oxidized readily. Both hemoglobin and carboxyhemoglobin dissolve readily in water. Carboxyhemoglobin is formed rapidly in the body during exposure to carbon monoxide. The result is a decreased transport capacity of the hemoglobin for oxygen.

Hemoglobin is found in the red blood cells of all vertebrates, including man. It is the oxygen carrier of blood. The combination of oxygen with hemoglobin forms oxyhemoglobin in a reversible reaction. The combination of carbon monoxide with hemoglobin forms carboxyhemoglobin. Hemoglobin has an affinity for carbon monoxide that is over 100 times its affinity of oxygen.

There is no single type of hemoglobin in human blood; at least twenty different kinds of human hemoglobin are known, each with an unique amino acid composition and specific physico-chemical characteristics (Diem, 1962).

Even nonsmokers have traces of carboxyhemoglobin in the blood. In heavy smokers, the carboxyhemoglobin may range from 6 to 8% of the total hemoglobin in the blood. This amount can rise to 12% in those persons who smoke excessively for the better part of a day.

Brief respiration of air rich in carbon monoxide followed by up to 6 hours of breathing a more dilute mixture maintains a blood level of 15% carboxyhemoglobin in an experimental subject lying down at a simulated altitude of 15,000 feet. A heavy smoker was exposed to these conditions; he began at a level of 6.8% carboxyhemoglobin and soon went up to 15%. He denied symptoms during the first hour. After that time, headache occurred and became progressively more severe. There was growing and continual nausea, mental confusion, restlessness, pallor, cold extremities, and a state of mild shock. These symptoms heightened with time. The blood carboxyhemoglobin held close to 15%.

A second subject at 10,000 feet simulated altitude (the elevation of Leadville, Colorado) and having 15% carboxyhemoglobin reported escalating headache and recurring nausea in the course of the closing hours of exposure, despite his combined arterial oxygen and carbon monoxide saturation of 97%.

At sea level with nearly complete blood saturation with oxygen and carbon monoxide, an experienced physiologist maintained that a short exposure causing a 30% carboxyhemoglobin is dangerous, especially if the subject is exercising (Rowan and Coleman, 1962).

One method of treating carbon monoxide poisoning involves forcing the victim to breathe pure oxygen through a mask under pressure twice that at sea level. The carbon monoxide is washed out of the blood rapidly under these conditions. Observations on patients so treated are useful in evaluating the toxic action of carbon monoxide. A pair of interesting and informative cases follow.

A female nineteen years old was rushed in for treatment of carbon monoxide poisoning. She was breathing without external aid; her reflexes were all present. She could be aroused with difficulty; her responses were minimal. She would have been unable to make the necessary responses to save her life if a hazardous situation arose. Her carboxyhemoglobin level upon arrival for treatment was 26%. Oxygen under pressure was successful in her rapid recovery.

A second case involved a forty-seven-year-old male who was brought in for treatment. He was in deep coma; color was ashen-gray; pupils of the eyes widely dilated; upper limbs spastic. No spontaneous breathing could be observed; no pulse. He would normally have been called moribund (not long for this world). His carboxyhemoglobin level was 50%. Oxygen under pressure helped him to survive the episode.

As a general rule, levels of carboxyhemoglobin of 15% or greater should be avoided, particularly if they are maintained for a long time during which the subject must be completely alert mentally. Table 6-II may be useful.

Table 6-II
TOXICITY TO MAN OF INHALED CARBON MONOXIDE IN AIR

Amount of CO in Air	Time of Action	Effect
1 percent	Few minutes	Death
1/20 of 1 percent	0.5 to 2 hours	Giddiness
1/10 of 1 percent	Short time	Inability to walk
1/5 of 1 percent	Short time	Unconsciousness
4/5 of 1 percent	Few minutes	Death

Mechanism of Toxic Action

Carbon monoxide in general is poisonous to man simply because it competes most successfully with oxygen for attachment points on the hemoglobin molecule. For every carbon monoxide molecule hooked to a hemoglobin position, one atom of oxygen is excluded. Until recently, all experimental evidence indicated that the toxic action of carbon monoxide stemmed exclusively from its formation of carboxyhemoglobin. There now is evidence that "carbon monoxide may have a direct toxic effect on the myocardium [heart muscle]" (Matthew and Lawson, 1975).

The poisoning action of carbon monoxide occurs in two stages. First, the various tissues and organs of the body in the person exposed to carbon monoxide become depleted of life-giving oxygen (they become anoxic). Very shortly after a victim is taken out of the poisonous atmosphere, the developing anoxia is usually reversed, and exposure to pure air in virtually all cases "washes out" the carbon monoxide.

However, if exposure to the carbon monoxide is prolonged, a second stage (often called *a vicious circle*) develops from the first stage. Figure 6-6 illustrates some of the critical occurrences of the second stage.

All victims of carbon monoxide poisoning must be judged as

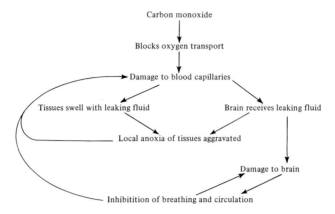

Figure 6-6. The vicious circle.

being in critical condition. Immediate first aid is mandatory:

1. Remove the victim to clean air.
2. Initiate cardiopulmonary resuscitation if needed.
3. Prevent the victim from absolutely all activity. Any physical action on the victim's part that might raise the body's oxygen requirement is harmful.
4. If pure medical oxygen is available it should be administered immediately to the victim once it is established that the victim is breathing spontaneously.
5. The victim must be given medical attention as speedily as can be arranged.

Some Responses to Carbon Monoxide Poisoning

A few hints on the responses and behavior of victims poisoned with carbon monoxide may be useful.

Older persons with hardening of the arteries are in graver danger than are younger individuals with efficient circulatory systems. Persons who have had a heart attack or a stroke or who suffer from a lung disease are critical "risks" if exposed to carbon monoxide.

At times, a carbon monoxide poisoned victim may be agitated, uncooperative, and even bordering on what appears to be hysteria.

These actions are signs of severe poisoning and suggest that the person is close to developing irreversible brain damage. These afflicted persons may show signs of a high fever.

Damage to the heart as a direct action of carbon monoxide has been seen more frequently recently. This kind of cardiac damage is signaled by fast, irregular heartbeat, severely lowered blood pressure, and shock. Pulmonary edema (fluid in the lungs) may occur and prevent adequate breathing. In emergency rooms, this condition is often treated by delivering oxygen under higher than atmospheric pressure. "Patients with moderate or severe carbon monoxide poisoning frequently have marked nausea, and vomiting and incontinence of faeces is common" (Matthew and Lawson, 1975).

The flushed, pink color of textbook cases of carbon monoxide poisoning is not always seen. If discoloration is present, one is safe in concluding that severe poisoning has occurred. If absent, one need not be surprised. Cold sweat is often observed.

Behavioral Effects

Carbon monoxide in low concentrations is known to reduce vigilance in those exposed to it. The performance of tasks that require an integration of time and motion estimates is decreased. The solving of complex problems seems unchanged (Weiss and Laties, 1975).

Studies have been made with volunteer males and females exposed to concentrations of carbon monoxide of 2, 50, 100, 200, and 500 ppm in air for up to 5 hours.

At lower concentrations (represented by a level of carboxyhemoglobin in the blood of 20% or less), there was no change in time perception. Likewise, there seemed to be no modification of manual coordination nor performance of arithmetic tasks under similar experimental conditions.

Smokers and nonsmokers react slightly differently to carbon monoxide exposure. The latter show impaired vigilance (in standardized tests) after breathing 111 ppm carbon monoxide in air, a level that raised the carboxyhemoglobin blood level to nearly 7%. Smokers, on the other hand, showed no change in vigilance after breathing 111 ppm carbon monoxide in air, a situation that raised their blood carboxyhemoglobin level to nearly 7%. The differences in responses between the two groups may represent physiological adjustment to higher base levels of carbon monoxide in the smoker group.

Animal Responses

One interesting study on animals concludes that exposure of several mammalian species to high levels of carbon monoxide in the air that they breathed (CO, 460 to 575 mg/cu. m. of air for 168 days) exerted no adverse effect on animal survival, rates of growth, nor clinical chemical values. Moreover, the exposure caused no pathological changes in the central nervous system (Theodore et al., 1971).

Human Experiments

In one experimental study of carbon monoxide poisoning in man, male volunteers were exposed to various high concentrations of carbon monoxide ranging from 1000 ppm for 10 minutes to 35,600 ppm for 45 seconds. The carbon monoxide was absorbed rapidly by the subjects, resulting in a marked change in blood carboxyhemoglobin concentration according to the following equation:

Change in % COHb/liter $= 1.036 \log$ (ppm CO inhaled) $- 4.4793$

Rapid increases in blood carboxyhemoglonin (COHb) saturation to 12% and 9% respectively brought about immediate frontal headache. Exposure to 35,600 ppm CO caused changes in the electrocardiogram within 20 seconds after exposure began; the changes persisted for 10 minutes after exposure to CO ended. No changes in brain function under any of the above conditions were observed (Stewart et al., 1973).

Guide for Poisoning Investigators

Police investigators and forensic science specialists who support the investigation must recognize that poisoning cases demand relatively technical procedures of investigation and a thoroughness that cannot be cut short without resulting disaster if the case gets into court (Wells, 1968, 1974).

An adequate investigation of a case of poisoning involves a minimum of three steps:

1. The poison must be isolated from the material available (human tissue, body fluids, stomach contents, or some unknown chemical substance). In some instances, a metabolite must be isolated because the human body converts the poison administered into another chemical species.
2. The extracted poison must be identified.
3. The total amount of poison in the victim must be estimated as precisely as possible. The value arrived at must then be compared with the lethal dose that is known.

Potentially toxic drugs and other chemicals found at the scene, on the person of the victim, in the clothing, purse, or other possession must be collected, labeled carefully, and brought as evidence to the laboratory toxicologist in whatever container the chemical was in at the scene. Often such a procedure can make or break a poisoning case.

Carbon Monoxide and Heart Disease

Data are now available in such quantity and of such quality (both clinical observation and experimental results) that there is no longer serious argument over the contention that carbon monoxide is the most deleterious component of tobacco smoke. There seems to be a harmful effect from carbon monoxide, in and of itself, on the heart and blood vessels (Roche, 1970). The elevation of serum cholesterol accompanies the regular intake of large amounts of CO.

The main physiological effects of carbon monoxide seem to be primarily related to the decreased oxygen in the tissues of the exposed individual. It is clear that CO inhalation interferes with oxygen transport by blood hemoglobin in two ways: (1) there is the carbon monoxide/hemoglobin reaction that prevents that portion of hemoglobin present as carboxyhemoglobin (COHb) from combining with oxygen; and (2) the presence of carboxyhemo-globin causes a leftward shift in the classic oxyhemoglobin dissociation curve, which at the tissue level means less oxygen available to cells, especially at low oxygen tensions. According to the *Smoking and Health Bulletin* of the Public Health Service, U.S. Department of Health, Education and Welfare (1970), carbon monoxide from tobacco smoke poses a clear, severe, and present danger to human beings.

Exposures to adequate environmental levels of CO increase COHb concentrations in human subjects. The amount of this increase is reasonably predictable and must be considered in relation to exposure to CO in inhaled cigarette smoke as well as to occupational and domestic exposures. The increase in body COHb results in some degree of impairment of tissue oxygenation. Exposure for 5 hours to between 10 and 12 ppm of CO has been shown to increase the COHb levels in nonsmokers by at least 0.5 percent. Such an increase adds appreciably to the body burden of COHb in those who do not already have such a body burden from cigarette smoking. Longer exposures could have produced a somewhat greater increase. The possible contribution of ambient community CO exposure to the mortality of persons hospitalized with myocardial infarction has been investigated. The evidence suggests that daily average CO values in excess of about 10 ppm may be associated with an increase in mortality in patients hospitalized with myocardial infarction. In two studies, persons driving motor vehicles that were involved in accidents had higher COHb levels than "control" populations. Possible mechanisms by which CO might affect the capability to drive a motor vehicle are suggested in the available data on CO effects upon visual sensitivity, psychological test performance, and accurate estimation of time intervals. Research to clarify uncertainty regarding the health effects of CO should include the relationship, if any, between ambient CO and COHb levels and the occurrence of motor vehicle accidents when weather and driving conditions, cigarette smoking, alcohol and drug use, and other factors are adjusted and controlled (Goldsmith and Cohen, 1969).

Additive Effects

Combinations of carbon monoxide and ethanol function additively, according to animal experiments (Pankow et al., 1974). Various combinations of ethanol and carbon monoxide administered to experimental animals at different time schedules, in single or in repeated exposures, all showed additive, not synergistic effects; high levels of one of the agents were necessary to demonstrate the action clearly. The point of these studies, in a practical sense, is that they sound a warning to automobile drivers, airplane pilots, tunnel guards, and others who might be exposed to carbon monoxide to be alert to the fact that alcohol in their blood may well aggravate the lethal situation. In questionable cases of alcohol deaths or carbon monoxide deaths, investigators might seriously consider carefully done blood tests for both of these toxic chemicals.

SOME EXAMPLES. The precise quantitative influence of carbon monoxide on human performance and comfort is still not worked out. It is known that for every ppm of carbon monoxide that gets into the alveoli of the lungs, 0.16 percent of the hemoglobin in the human body is put out of action (Foreman, 1962).

In the atmosphere, an extreme value of 93 ppm of carbon monoxide has been recorded. Values of 4 to 8 ppm are more usually encountered. The smoking of cigarettes demonstrably increases the carbon monoxide concentration in the surrounding air. Smokers who live in cities often show that 8 percent of their hemoglobin has been inactivated by carbon monoxide. If the carboxyhemoglobin (the compound formed by the combination of carbon monoxide and hemoglobin) concentration in the blood does not surpass 5%, individuals do not complain of illness or of not feeling well. If the carboxyhemoglobin content of the blood increases over 20%, signs and symptoms of carbon monoxide poisoning become moderately severe. Concentrations above 50% lead to unconsciousness and death. The usual complaints associated with carbon monoxide poisoning include anoxia, fatigue, dizziness, and headaches. Severe exposures to carbon monoxide bring on signs of damage to the nervous system: ataxia, twitching, and eventually coma (unconsciousness).

THE POISONED POLICEMAN. The question of chronic carbon monoxide poisoning is still debated among toxicologists. An interesting case comes to mind of a policeman who went through an episode suggesting reality of chronic carbon monoxide poisoning in certain circumstances.

The officer had been seen on and off for a number of years by his physician and in the hospital for unexplainable neurological (nervous system) and psychiatric (mental) signs and symptoms that clearly indicated that something was wrong with the individual. A careful review of his history, including a detailed analysis of his job assignments as well as a thorough clinical battery of tests, disclosed that he was exposed to high concentrations of carbon monoxide during his duty hours. At the time he was tested, his blood was 20% saturated with carbon monoxide. He was ordered on extended sick leave, at the expense of the department. After several months, the odd signs and symptoms disappeared. The excessive carbon monoxide in the blood had disappeared also. The officer was returned to duty in a completely new assignment (one that insured a minimal exposure to carbon monoxide); the signs and symptoms did not return. The officer eventually made the rank of sergeant.

The case in question supports the view that carbon monoxide may persist in the body for several weeks after exposure to the toxic gas ceases. The precise manner in which the tie-up of the carbon monoxide occurs in the body is not clear. It does seem, however, that prolonged exposure to high levels of carbon monoxide in some individuals results in the long-term storing of the toxicant in the body—possibly by combination with myoglobin (the red coloring matter in muscle chemically related to hemoglobin), which then functions as a slow-release reservoir of carbon monoxide into the blood (Foreman, 1962).

Environmental Carbon Monoxide

Carbon monoxide is probably the most plentiful and extensively disseminated pollutant in the lower atmosphere. One view is that the origin of atmospheric carbon monoxide is principally from human activities. According to this contention, about 63 percent of the carbon monoxide that is injected into the atmosphere from human technological endeavors comes from the burning of fossil fuels in motor vehicles. It is further maintained that 7 percent of the total carbon monoxide in the atmosphere derives from natural sources such as swamps, volcanos, and forest fires.

The amount of carbon monoxide in the atmosphere varies from place to place in a significant way. Diurnal, weekly, and seasonal variations in carbon monoxide content of the atmosphere are the usual condition.

Recall that the combination of carbon monoxide with hemoglobin reduces the capacity of the hemoglobin to carry oxygen. Moreover, the presence of carbon monoxide on the hemoglobin molecule prevents the usually ready release to the bodily tissues of the already decreased amount of oxygen that is still carried by the hemoglobin.

As a result, if a person has 5 percent of his hemoglobin saturated with carbon monoxide, he is in a physiological state equal to being at an altitude of 8,000 to 10,000 feet (about 2400 to 3000 m). The effects can be illustrated by changes in visual sensitivity.

Carbon Monoxide Saturation (%)	Visual Sensitivity (Altitude Equivalent Feet)
5	8,000-10,000
15	15,000-19,000 (4500 to 5700 m)

OTHER TOXIC INHALANTS

Cyanide

Cyanide in the form of the gas hydrocyanic acid (HCN) is used for fumigating. It also is used in the metal-plating industry and in gold mining. The fatal oral dose of cyanide is 0.05 gm. Individuals exposed to cyanide show rapid responses to the chemical, which prevents the various tissues of the body from using oxygen that is delivered by the blood. The action is so rapid that as a general rule, first aid is futile. Artificial respiration may work, although adequate oxygen in the blood will not reverse the poisoning simply because the tissues cannot use the oxygen even though it is supplied in large amounts. There are some special chemical kits that contain methemoglobin formers. If these antidotes can be administered soon enough, there is some hope that the victim might be saved. The only effective treatment of hydrocyanic acid poisoning is prevention. Table 6-III gives toxicological information for a number of noxious gases encountered by modern man.

Fluorocarbons Can Harm

A peculiar class of chemicals called fluoroalkanes is used as fire-extinguishing agents, refrigerants, and solvents. Some of these fluorocarbons are found in general household and drug preparations as aerosol propellants. These same chemicals are used in a harmful way by "sniffers" who apparently obtain some sort of kick from the toxic effects of inhaling the vapors. Probably the anesthetic action of most of these agents is the basis for the sniffer's kick. Indeed, one of the chemicals in this class is used as a surgical anesthetic in veterinary and human operations.

Fluoroalkanes are poisonous to human beings under certain conditions. They enter the human body through the respiratory organs. Their toxicity is relatively low. However, if the materials are used carelessly in enclosed spaces or are frankly abused by inhaling for kicks. damage to the brain and the cardiovascular system (heart and blood vessels) can occur.

The action on the brain by these inhalants results in changes in perception, lengthening of the reaction time, and decreased ability to concentrate on complex tasks of an intellectual nature. These effects occur when the subjects breath 10 to 15% trifluorobromomethane ($CBrF_3$), for example, in air.

The action of these chemicals on the heart is of concern because they upset the normal blood pressure relationships in the heart by depressing the contractility of the heart muscle. The heart also shows arrythmias such as extra beats, missed beats, and palpitations. The electrical activity of the heart is modified by exposure to fluoroalkanes. The adverse effects on the brain almost always occur before the effects on the heart.

Exposure to these chemicals, in excess, poses a life threat to the subject because of the altered responsiveness he has to his surroundings.

The first aid procedure for treating poisonings from these agents is simple. Remove the victim from the source of exposure; insure that the victim is breathing spontaneously in a noncontaminated atmosphere. If the victim is not breathing, use the mouth-to-mouth procedure until emergency services are available. Do not permit the victim to engage in any physical activity other than lying quietly until competent medical personnel take over (Back and Van Stee, 1977).

Chlorine

This inhalant is an irritant gas greenish yellow in color. Its specific gravity is about 2.5 times that of air. Hence, it tends to drop to the lower parts of an enclosed space and will creep into depressions and the like. It is readily liquified. Commercially, it is carried in the typical compressed gas cylinder or in tank cars on railroads or tank trailers on trucks.

Chlorine is used as a disinfectant (in city water supplies, for example), in metal technology, in the textile industry and other industries as a bleach, and in the food industry.

It is about 20 times as poisonous as hydrogen chloride. Acting by abstracting hydrogen from moist tissues of the body, it releases oxygen and combines with the released hydrogen to form hydrochloric acid. Thus it is that chlorine, which was used as a chemical warfare agent by the Germans in World War I, exerts its damaging action by oxidation (through release of oxygen) and irritation that is caused by the hydrochloric acid formed from the chlorine and hydrogen abstracted from the body tissues.

In very low concentration, chlorine has been reported to serve prophylactically against respiratory infections. Practically, it is entirely too dangerous to be used for such a purpose. A brief exposure to 1000 ppm chlorine in air is lethal to man and large animals.

The signs of chlorine poisoning include: lacrimation (tear formation), rhinorrhea (nasal discharge), salivation, coughing, vomiting, and syncope (fainting). It may take an hour or more for all the signs to develop.

The first treatment is removal of the victim from the chlorine atmosphere. Oxygen should then be administered by mask for as long as needed. In many cases, oxygen was required for 96 hours after the exposure to chlorine. Under hospital conditions, oxygen administered under elevated pressure is highly recommended. Antibiotics are frequently given in order to prevent pneumonia.

There is no evidence that tuberculosis or chronic lung disease results from exposure to chlorine.

Anesthetic Deaths

At times the forensic toxicologist is asked to investigate an anesthetic death. Much of this work involves gas chromatography.

There is a case reported in which a patient died because a tank of nitrous oxide, an effective anesthetic gas, was contaminated with other oxides of nitrogen that are poisonous.

In most cases of this sort, interpretation must be cautious. Indeed, if the amount of unknown material available is inadequate for testing, the toxicologist should refuse to perform any analyses. If, under the conditions, he is forced to analyze inadequate samples, he then should refuse to render an opinion.

Carbon Tetrachloride

This volatile substance is found in some home dry-cleaning, spot-removing, or rug-cleaning preparations. It is also found in fire extinguisher fluids. If the concentration of carbon tetrachloride in air builds up to 50 ppm or more, it becomes dangerous to man. Diagnosis of poisoning is usually made on the basis of attending circumstances and the peculiar pungent odor of the chemical on the victim's breath or clothing.

Carbon tetrachloride is a potent damaging chemical to the liver and kidneys. The destructive effect may be delayed from 3 to 10 days after exposure if the victim lives that long. In acute poisonings, the substance has an anesthetic effect. First aid involves removal of the victim from the source of exposure; artificial respiration is administered if necessary; oxygen is given by mask if available. Medical treatment must be instituted without delay. Hospital emergency personnel should be clearly informed what poison was involved, if known, so that treatment to prevent brain, liver, and kidney damage can be initiated.

Petroleum Distillates

These volatile substances are frequently found in insecticide sprays and similar aerosol preparations. Many of them are more poisonous than the pesticide itself. A gasoline– or kerosenelike odor helps to diagnose the problem in unconscious victims. Labeled containers of the material in the vicinity are informative.

Removal from the source of exposure, artificial respiration if needed, and oxygen by mask if available are the first aid measures to take. Medical treatment must be insured.

Nitrous Oxide

Nitrous oxide gas is a mild anesthetic and an effective analgesic (pain-killing) agent (DiMaio and Garriott, 1978). It is used almost exclusively in dental surgery. In the 1800s, it was used at parties because inhaling it gave pleasant side-effects—hence its name "laughing gas."

From 1958 to 1978, there was a single record of death published in the English language medical literature from abuse of nitrous oxide. Four deaths were reported in 1978 from its abuse. "Nitrous oxide is an extremely safe gas, even when used without medical supervision" (DiMaio and Garriott, 1978). Under peculiar circumstances, nitrous oxide can cause death, but historically the incidence of such deaths is negligible. Legislation at any level of government to "curb abuse" of nitrous oxide by people is frivolous.

Gas chromatography can be used effectively for demonstrating nitrous oxide from lung air and in blood after suitable pretreatment. Blood nitrous oxide concentrations from the four recent fatalities varied from 5 to 9 ml/dl of blood. The nitrous oxide in the lung air of the dead victims varied from 14 to 23%; the oxygen amounted to 5 to 13% in the same lung air samples.

Abuse of Volatile Substances

Fortunately, the wave of popularity for *glue sniffing,* a term used loosely for the activity of inhaling a variety of volatile substances in order to get a kick, seems to have passed. The mild epidemic of inhaling volatile materials, especially by adolescents, seems to have plateaued at a comparatively low level.

Some rather foolish laws and ordinances were passed in order to "control" the epidemic; these actions were taken by adults who should have known better but who opted to behave in an adolescent fashion. The decrease in the sniffing activity probably came about, not as a result of ill-conceived laws of "thou shall not," but rather from low-key dissemination of the facts about the permanent damage to the human body resulting from such sniffing of toxic materials. Truthful information (*all* the truth) presented in a noninflammatory way and documented in a sober fashion has a persuasive effect on young Americans. On the other hand, the iron fist seems not to work.

The following list of references should be of help to law enforcement personnel who may be responsible for disseminating information to parents, politicians, young adults, and others concerning abuse of volatile substances (Ronaghan, 1972).

Table 6-III
TOXICOLOGICAL INFORMATION ON NOXIOUS GASES*

Gas	Biological Action	Maximum Acceptable Concentration	Sensitivity of Determination
Ammonia	Tissue corrosion; death	50 ppm	3 ppm
Arsine	Headache; organ damage; death	0.05 ppm	0.05 ppm
Carbon dioxide	Unconsciousness; death	5000 ppm	120 ppm
Carbonyl sulfide	Irritant; respiratory paralysis	@ 20 ppm	—
Chlorine	Lung irritation; death	1 ppm	—
Chlorine dioxide	bronchitis; unconsciousness; death	0.1 ppm	0.15 ppm

Table 6-III
TOXICOLOGICAL INFORMATION ON NOXIOUS GASES (*Continued*)

Gas	*Biological Action*	*Maximum Acceptable Concentration*	*Sensitivity of Determination*
Cyanogen chloride	Respiratory irritation	<0.5 ppm	1 ppm
Fluorine	Irritation of all moist tissues; spasm of larynx	0.1 ppm	—
Hydrogen chloride	Erosion of tissues; irritation of eyes and respiratory tract	5 ppm	1 ppm
Hydrogen cyanide	Paralysis of respiration; death	10 ppm	1 ppm
Hydroen fluoride	Severe irritation to tissues	3 ppm	20 μgm
Hydrogen silenide	Pneumonitis; death	0.05 ppm	—
Hydrogen sulfide	Headache; respiratory paralysis; death	10 ppm	1 ppm
Hydrogen telluride	destruction of blood cells	0.05 ppm	—
Nitrogen dioxide	Irritant to lungs; delayed deaths	5 ppm	—
Nitrosyl chloride	Much like phosphene	100 ppm lethal	—
Ozone	Headache; pulmonary edema; hemorrhage; no known deaths	0.1 ppm	—
Phosphine	Nausea; breathing distress; pulmonary edema; delayed deaths	0.3 ppm	0.02 ppm
Stibine (SbH_3)	Blood and liver damage	0.1 ppm	—
Sulfur dioxide	Tissue irritant; chronic bronchitis	5 ppm	1 ppm
Ethyl amine Methyl amine	Irritant to respiratory system	10 ppm	—
Ethylene oxide	Headache; kidney damage; narcosis	50 ppm	—
Formaldehyde	Respiratory irritant	5 ppm	0.5 ppm
Methyl bromide	Headache; dizziness; tremors; central nervous system damage; delayed deaths	20 ppm	—

Table 6-III
TOXICOLOGICAL INFORMATION ON NOXIOUS GASES *(Continued)*

Gas	Biological Action	Maximum Acceptability Concentration	Sensitivity of Determination
Methyl chloride	Mental confusion; coma; death	100 ppm	—
Monochloroethylene	Tissue irritant	500 ppm	—
Fluorocarbons	Mild narcosis	1000 ppm; 100 ppm for CBr_2F_2	—
Ketene	Exceedingly toxic; similar to phosphine	0.5 ppm	—
Phosgene	World War I poison gas; pulmonary edema; death from anoxia and cardiac failure	0.1 ppm	0.5 ppm with test paper

*As a result of federal laws, various "standards" have been set for the amounts of toxic gases in air. If legal matters are involved, the Federal Register must be consulted or the Environmental Protection Agency queried for specific legal "standards." This table gives scientific values based on the best available technical data; no assumption must be made concerning the legal weight of the data (Look, 1966).

Volatile Substances References

Ackerly, W.C., Gibson, G.: Lighter fluid sniffing. *Am J Psychiatry, 120(11):* 1056-1061, 1964.

Adey, W.R.: The sense of smell. In Magoun, H.W. et al.: *Handbook of Physiology: A Critical Comprehensive Presentation of Physiological Knowledge and Concepts. Section 1. Neurophysiology, Vol. 1.* Washington, D.C. American Physiological Society, 1969, pp. 535-548.

Barker, G.H., Adams, W.T.: Glue sniffers. *Sociol Soc Res, 47(3):*298-310, 1963.

Brozovsky, M., Winkler, E.G.: Glue sniffing in children and adolescents. *NY State J Med, 65(15):*1984-1989, 1965.

Clinger, O.W., Johnson, N.A.: Purposeful inhalation of gasoline vapors. *Psychiatr Q, 25(4):*557-567, 1951.

Dodds, J., Santostefano, S.: A comparison of the cognitive functioning of glue-sniffers and non-sniffers. *J Pediatr, 64(4):*565-570, 1964.

Easson, W.M.: Gasoline addiction in children. *Pediatrics, 29(2):*250-254, 1962.

Friedman, P.: Some observations on the sense of smell. *Psychoanal Q, 28(3):*307-329, 1959.

Glaser, H.G., Massengale, O.N.: Glue sniffing in children. *JAMA, 181(4):* 300-303, 1962.

Jacobziner, H., Raybin, H.W.: Lead poisoning and glue sniffing intoxication. *NY State J Med, 63(19):*2846-2848, 1963.

Lawton, J.J. Jr., Malmquist, C.P.: Gasoline addiction in children. *Phychiatr Q, 35(3):*555-561, 1961.

Macmillan, W.L. Jr.: The scent of danger. *The Police Chief, 20(5):*42-44, 1963.

Massengale, O.N., et al.: Physical and psychologic factors in glue sniffing. *N Engl J Med, 269(16):*1340-1344, 1963.

Pierson, H.W.: Glue sniffing, a hazardous hobby. *J Sch Health, 34(5):*252-255, 1964.

Press, E., Done, A.K.: Solvent sniffing physiologic effects and community control measures for intoxication from the intentional inhalation of organic solvents. Part I. *Pediatrics, 39(3):*451-461, 1967.

Press, E., Done, A.K.: Solvent sniffing physiologic effects and community control measures for intoxication from the intentional inhalation of organic solvents. Part III. *Pediatrics, 39(4):*611-622, 1967.

Rubin, T., Babbs, J.: The glue sniffer. *Federal Probation, 34(3):*23-28, 1970.

Taylor, G.J., Harris, W.S.: Glue sniffing causes heart block in mice. *Science, 170(19):*866-868, 1970.

Warning Against Deliberate Misuse of Aerosol Products. New York, Aerosol Education Bureau, 1969.

Will Death Come Without Warning? New York, Aerosol Education Bureau, 1969.

Winick, C.: Teenage glue sniffers reported in many areas. *Social Health News, 37(9):*1-2, 1962.

Winick, C., Goldstein, J.: *The Glue Sniffing Problem.* New York, American Social Health Association, 1965.

Chapter 7

POLICE RIOT CONTROL CHEMICALS

THIS CHAPTER concerns itself with the toxicological or poisonous effects of the several nonlethal chemicals that exert peculiar biological effects on human beings so that they are rendered temporarily incapable of engaging in aggressive activity. Two of these chemical agents are primarily used by police to aid in quelling a riot or to subdue a violent individual without harm (Swearingen, 1966).

The chapter makes no pretense at outlining the tactical use of riot control agents, nor does it concern itself, other than incidentally, with hardware for disseminating such agents. The goal of this chapter is to inform law enforcement personnel about the biological action of these chemicals on man as well as to suggest methods for alleviating (by decontamination or therapy) the distress caused by the agents when such first aid is appropriate.

What Are Riot Control Agents?

Chemicals used for riot control or to subdue violent individuals are, in general, substances that in small amounts produce local irritation. The action usually centers on vulnerable surfaces of the body such as eyes, nasal passages, and mouth. If the concentration of the chemical is great enough, irritating effects occur in the upper part of the respiratory system or on the skin; with some agents in this general group, nausea and vomiting may develop.

Although these chemicals are at times referred to as gases (tear gas, vomiting gas), they are solid chemicals dispersed in the air in the form of an extremely fine dust or an aerosol. The two most

common chemicals for riot control use by police are chloroacetophenone, referred to by the military code CN, and orthochlor-
benzylidenemalononitrile, code symbol CS.

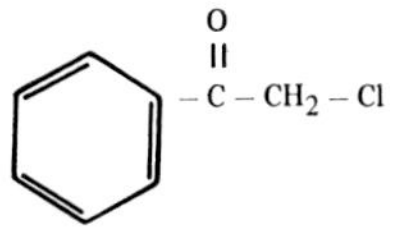

O
||
$-C-CH_2-Cl$

Chemical structure of CN

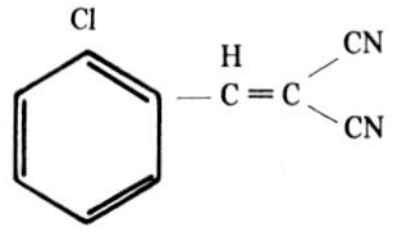

Cl

$-C=C<^{CN}_{CN}$ (H)

Chemical structure of CS

Kinds of Riot Control Chemicals

There are a number of irritating chemicals that are available
for riot control. The following list includes virtually all the "tear
gas" chemicals known.

Ethylbromoacetate, $CH_2BrCOOC_2H_5$
Chloroacetone, CH_3COCH_2Cl
Xylyl bromide, $C_6H_4CH_3CH_2Br$
Benzyl bromide, $C_6H_5CH_2Br$
Bromoacetone, CH_3COCH_2Br
Bromomethylethylketone, $BrCH_2COCH_2CH_3$
Iodoacetone, CH_3COCH_2I
Ethyliodoacetate, $CH_2ICOOC_2H_5$
Benzyliodide, $C_6H_5CH_2I$
Acrolein, CH_2CHCHO
Cyanogen bromide, $CNBr$
Chloropicrin, CCl_3NO
Phenylcarbylamine chloride, $C_6H_5CNCl_2$
Bromobenzylcyanide, $C_6H_5CHBrCN$
Capsaicin, $C_{18}H_{27}NO_2$
Chloroacetophenone, $C_6H_5COCH_2Cl$ (code designation is
CN)

In addition, there are various mixtures of lacrimating agents that have found limited use in police work. The relatively new agent, orthochlorobenzylidenemalononitrile, code designation CS, $ClC_6H_4CHC(CN)_2$, is a general irritating agent. Its reputation in riot control is excellent.

Chloroacetophenone

During World War I, chloroacetophenone (CN) was investigated in the United States, where the technological prerequisites for its industrial production were in existence. It was not used in that war, since the production plants were still under construction at the end of the war.

During World War II, bromoacetophenone and chloroacetophenone were manufactured in great quantities in all the belligerent states. Apart from their possible military use, most of these substances were and still are used as police weapons in the capitalist countries. Since bromoacetophenone and chloroacetophenone have the same properties, it is sufficient to limit the discussion here to chloroacetophenone as the most important representative of the group.

There are several methods for preparing chloroacetophenone chemically; all give the same pure effective product. Chloroacetophenone can be produced in the laboratory or in industrial lots. The agent itself is a colorless, crystalline substance that melts at 57° to 58°C. The industrial product is gray in color, probably as a result of harmless impurities.

Although the vapor pressure of chloroacetophenone is relatively low, the volatility as 20° C amounting to 0.11 mg/liter and the attenuation factor for volatility in the field being taken at a maximum value of 10^{-2}, the vapor pressure is adequate to make a terrain contaminated with chloroacetophenone impassable without protective masks. The threshold for detectable chloroacetophenone symptoms is 5×10^{-4} mg/liter.

The effect of chloroacetophenone vapors is dependent on the outside temperature. The volatility below 10°C is too low for an effective concentration to develop. It is possible, nevertheless, to use it in cold weather in the form of an aerosol. Chloroacetophenone is sufficiently stable with respect to heat and can therefore be used not only in shells and hand grenades, but also in low-temperature carbonation gases. It is principally used as an aerosol warfare agent.

The fact that chloroacetophenone does not decompose at its own boiling point makes it possible to pour the liquid product directly into shells and to mix it with low-carbonation mixtures, even with explosives, for example, 2,4,6-trinitrotoluene, especially as these have approximately the same specific gravity.

Chloroacetophenone is probably insoluble in water but dissolves well in the usual organic solvents, such as chloralkanes, alkanoles, and benzene. It dissolves in certain proportions in some chemical warfare agents such as sulfur mustard, phosgene, trichloronitromethane, and cyanogen chloride.

Chloroacetophenone is by structure a mixed aliphatic-aromatic ketone. As such, it is relatively stable and slow to react. The well-known reaction of the aliphatic ketones with the carbonyl reagents such as hydroxyl amine and hydrazine occurs here also. On the other hand, no hydrogen sulfite additive compound is formed.

Depending on the density of poisoning and the local and meteorological conditions, chloroacetophenone solutions may persist for hours and days. Chloroacetophenone-chloropicrin solution mixed with trichloronitromethane is said to have a persistency in the woods of 2 hours in the summer and up to a week in the winter. In the open, 1 hour in the summer and 6 hours in the winter is counted on.

The thermal stability of chloroacetophenone is good. It is stable when detonated. It is only when exposed to a temperature above 300°C for at least 15 minutes that it breaks down noticeably. Even in boiling water, chloroacetophenone is not hydrolyzed, or at least not noticeably so. Chloroacetophenone on the ground does not lose its properties even under a covering of snow. After the snow melts, it is again physiologically effective under correspondingly favorable temperatures. The same situation applies to chloroacetophenone poured into the ground.

The rate of hydrolysis is accelerated by alkalies. It is so slow at normal temperatures that this reaction is worthless for decontamination. A quantitative conversion is achieved only by boiling in alkali hydroxide solution, especially when alcoholic solutions are concerned. As a product of hydrolysis, oxymethylphenylketone (oxyacetophenone) is formed; the crystals of this product melt at 85°C.

Chloroacetophenone is not affected by atmospheric oxygen. In suitable solvents such as benzene and dioxane, chloroacetophenone is oxidized by powerful oxidizing agents such as chromic acid, sodium permanganate, and selenium dioxide hypochloride into benzene dicarboxylic acid. Phenylacetic acid and phenylglyoxal, as well as other substances, develop as by-products. Nitric acid sometimes has an oxidizing and sometimes a nitrifying effect on chloroacetophenone.

Under suitable conditions, further chlorination of the acetophenone is possible both in the side chain and in the nucleus. These chlorine derivatives have a slight eye-irritant effect but are more distinguished for their powerful skin-irritant effect. They have been considered for chemical warfare agents several times for that reason but have not been adopted.

The eye irritants such as chloroacetophenone have practically no military tactically exploitable toxicant effect, with the exception of those compounds mentioned in other groups of chemical warfare agents. After reaching the lower sensory threshold, they cause rather marked eye irritation. Some substances also have a certain skin-irritant effect even at low concentrations. Although this reaction is felt as very unpleasant, it is to be regarded as secondary. From the physiological point of view, chloroacetophenone has a threshold of 3×10^{-4} mg/liter. The tolerance limit is 2×10^{-3} mg/liter. It causes skin rashes on the face at 2×10^{-3} mg/liter.

The chemical formula of this agent is $C_6H_5COCH_2Cl$; it has a molecular weight of 154.59. The solid chemical melts at a temperature of 57° to 58° C (135° to 136° F). The boiling point of CN is 244° to 245° C (471° to 473° F). The chemical does not break down nor decompose with increased temperature up to the boiling point, nor does it readily decompose in water. When it does break down in water (hydrolyze), the products are hydrochloric acid and hydroxymethylphenylketone. The shelf-life is long. Metals exposed to CN may become tarnished. The agent has a smell that resembles apple blossoms.

CN is still used widely among police agencies around the world. One characteristic of CN that makes it attractive to police is the fact that "it is almost impossible to achieve a lethal concentration with CN" (Swearingen, 1966). Furthermore, "The suitability of CN as an agent for civil use has been proven many times over since the tear gas industry was established." Finally, Swearingen contends that "individuals exposed to CN vapors do not normally require any first aid, except to be removed to uncontaminated air and stand facing into the wind with their eyes open."

Toxicity of CN

This chemical was first synthesized in 1869 by a German scientist and is extensively used as a lacrimator (tear gas) by police around the world.

As a potent irritant of the eyes and the upper portions of the human respiratory system, within a matter of seconds after exposure to CN, the subject experiences a copious and uncontrollable flood of tears. If concentrations of CN in the air are great enough, the skin may be irritated, especially if it is moist. A few cases of nausea have been reported after exposures to especially heavy concentrations of CN. There has been reported an occasional allergic type of reaction, which seemed to be local and not systemic, in persons receiving a heavy dose of the agent concentrated over a small area of skin.

A CN concentration of 0.3 ml/cu. m. of air is the minimal effective level for this agent. A concentration of 5 to 10 mg/cu. m. of air is needed for optimal effects on man.

It is doubtful that a lethal concentration of CN could be produced out of doors. The concentration of CN needed to kill (be lethal to) 50 percent of the persons exposed is 10,000 mg-min./cu. m. This value, LC_{50}, would result from breathing for 10 minutes air concentrated with 100 mg (1 gm or $1/28$th of an ounce) of CN.

The Director of Public Health of Berkeley, California, made a medical evaluation of CN in the form of Chemical Mace® in response to a request from the city manager for such a study (Leonard, 1968). Dr. Leonard's report is given here *in extenso* because of its excellence and because it is directly related to the toxicity of riot control agents used by municipal police.

Use of Mace

As requested by City Council, I have carefully reviewed the material on Chemical Mace submitted by Dr. Stuart Frank of the Medical Committee for Human Rights. In addition, I have studied the relevant reports of the Surgeon General and the University of Michigan Medical School, and have read scientific papers and correspondence prepared by Dr. Lawrence Rose, Dr. Walter Byers, and others, and have discussed the subject of Chemical Mace with Dr. Rose, Dr. Byers, and with Dr. Thomas Milby, chief of the Bureau of Occupational Health of the California State Health Department.

In the material thus made available to this office there is a substantial body of objective factual data upon which all well-informed persons agree. In addition, there is an area of discussion based on inferences drawn from the objective data and on speculation based upon general biologic principles; in this area, dealing with the *potential* undesirable side effects of Mace, different authorities place different emphasis— some tending to minimize the potential damage and some tending to accentuate it. I believe a balanced judgment between the two extreme viewpoints (i.e., (1) Mace is completely innocuous, or (2) Mace is too dangerous to permit its use) presents the most constructive approach to the subject. The reasons for this belief are set forth below.

I. The basic facts are:

    A. The active ingredient in Chemical Mace is the same chemical as in tear gas. It is delivered from a pressurized cannister in a solvent mixture at a concentration of .9% to 1.2%.

    B. The active ingredient causes acute local tissue irritation, most commonly of the skin, eyes, and mucous membranes of the nose and throat.

    C. The longer the material is in contact with tissue, the more severe is the resulting irritation.

    D. The mixture of chemicals in the solvent and propellant are present in quantities and concentration well below the standards accepted for safety in industrial exposures, according to the Bureau of Occupational Health in the State Department of Public Health.

E. About 125 persons have been seen at Highland Hospital Emergency Room following exposure to Mace. According to Dr. Byers, careful follow-up by the ophthalmology service of the hospital has revealed no permanent eye injury.

F. Dr. Rose has seen twelve cases in San Francisco with lesions as follows: Nine had chemical burns of the cornea which subsided in 48 to 72 hours. Three had more persistent lesions of the eye, but recovered vision completely in 2 to 3 weeks. One of these has a small residual corneal scar that does not interfere with vision. Four of the twelve persons had second-degree skin burns of the face, including blistering and peeling. All healed with no permanent residual effects. Four had mental confusion and anxiety lasting one to two hours.

It is important to note that in each of these twelve cases the Mace was used in a manner that all authorities consider improper. It was used at a very short distance from the subject (6 in. to 2 ft.) and there was no post-exposure irrigation or other immediate treatment.

G. In 1967, the State Department of Public Health received reports of 22 policemen and one fireman in California having incurred injuries from Mace (14), Peacemaker (2), or similar devices, the type not stated (7). These reports come to the State Health Department as reports of industrial injuries under Workmen's Compensation. The injuries were either skin burns and/or conjunctivitis, with time lost from work varying from no lost time in 17 cases to a maximum of 7 days lost in one case. Some of the injuries occurred while subduing prisoners, some in training, and at least one from a leaking Mace cannister.

H. The Berkeley Police Department has developed standing orders and policies regarding precautions to be taken in the use of Mace. The Health Department reviewed these and made some suggestions for increased safeguards, which were subsequently incorporated into the Police Department's policies.

The above information is fairly clear and I believe there is general agreement regarding those facts.

II. This section attempts to summarize the major inferences and speculations upon which there are few "hard data" and which represent an area of honest differences of judgment among competent observers.

A. "Tear gas, delivered in ways other than as Mace, has produced permanent eye damage." Such damage has most commonly occurred with the use of the so-called "tear gas pen." With this device there is a blast that is produced by an explosive charge and the eye may be injured by a combination of the shock force, fragments of wadding, metallic fragments, or by solid particles of the tear gas itself being forced into the eye under great pressure. In my opinion, these cases of injury are of doubtful relevance to the problem under discussion because Chemical Mace is delivered as an aerosol under far less pressure and unaccompanied by solid particles or by explosive force.

B. "Tear gas may have a selective neurotoxic potential." This concern that tear gas may injure nerve tissue derives from chemical studies and clinical observations of anesthesia of the fingers that has occurred following accidental discharge of tear gas pens in people's hands. More basic biochemical research is needed in order to clarify the point. However, as in "A" above, this problem is not highly relevant to the major issues concerning Mace since dosage and mode of delivery of Mace are so different (less penetrating of tissue) from the reported cases of suspected nerve damage.

C. "The solvents found in Mace, alone or in combination, may produce systemic damage." To date, there is no evidence to support this hypothesis. One of the chemicals in the solvent, methyl chloroform, is quite toxic in concentrations above 500 parts per million. However, the concentration of methyl chloroform resulting from use of Mace is far below the toxic level.

D. "Casual and careless use of the material, stemming from the belief that it is completely innocuous, can cause damage." This is undoubtedly true. Like most toxic biologic reactions, as the time-dose exposure increases, the resulting body damage increases. Therefore, the material must be considered a *potent* part of the law enforcement arsenal, to be used with as much care and prudence as any other weapon.

E. "Persons with poor reflexes, or with cardiovascular disease may be more severely affected than otherwise healthy people." This is probably true and is consistent with general observations regarding response to any biologic stress. It is a problem to be considered in all situations where force is applied, whether the force is by means of a chemical agent such as Mace or a physical agent such as a baton. Which force is biologically more stressful in any given situation is a matter of individual judgment that must be based upon intelligent assessment of the unique circumstances in each situation.

F. "The ill effects of many chemicals (such as beryllium and the chemicals in cigarette smoke) take years or decades to develop, and this could be the case with Mace." This *possibility* cannot be denied. However, the same can be said of hundreds of synthetic chemicals in our modern environment, and there is little reason for Mace to be unusually suspect in this regard. The problem of long-term effects of new drugs and chemicals is one that is almost unavoidable in a rapidly changing technological society.

III. After consideration of the facts and inferences outlined above, it is clear that Chemical Mace is a potent product of current technology. Like most other new technical developments it has potential for constructive social usage, i.e., when employed correctly it can be used for society's benefit in intelligent law enforcement with minimal risk. However, like most other new technologies, it also has a potential for misuse, in which case it can be medically and socially harmful. Therefore, I believe that:

1) At this stage of our knowledge, the most rational posture to adopt is mid-way between the extreme views that Mace is either: a) completely innocuous and harmless or, b) its potential for damage is too great to ever permit its use.

2) At all times Mace should be viewed as a potential weapon whose use must be carefully regulated.

3) With *proper and prudent* use, the danger of serious or permanent damage from this weapon is minimal. With improper use (too close to the person, person lacking normal reflexes, in a closed space), or delay in post-exposure treatment, the hazard increases sharply.

4) As with all other weapons, the persons employing it must be thoroughly trained and supervised in its use and related limitations.

5) As with all other weapons, the relative hazard must be balanced against the relative value in law enforcement."

Eye Irritation

According to the Department of the Army (1966), CN or chloroacetophenone, the active agent in one form of Mace, causes severe eye irritation and some mild skin irritation; the effect is virtually instantaneous and results in severe lacrimation (production of tears). CS or orthochlorobenzylidenemalononitrile is a highly irritating but otherwise nontoxic incapacitating agent. Its action is instantaneous. Recovery is complete after removal of the exposed subject from the source of exposure. Rarely and only in extremely hazardous situations should Mace be used at a distance of less than 24 inches.

Dermatitis

Scattered cases of contact dermatitis caused by chloroacetophenone (CN) have been reported (Penneys, 1971). The agent can sensitize human beings, that is, make some people allergic to subsequent exposures. Some research workers suggest that CN is a "potent allergic sensitizer." The time necessary to bring on an allergic reaction to CN in the form of Mace, for example, is three to four minutes of contact with the chemical. Thorough washing of the exposed area with water (and soap if the eyes are avoided) may do much to circumvent the development of dermatitis if the washing is done within a few minutes after exposure to CN.

Some Practical Suggestions

CN in the form of Mace should be used after it becomes apparent that no other reasonable method will control a violent individual. After Mace is used, the parts of the body exposed to it should be flooded with water. Adequate washing of the eyes with a soft stream of water is the best and only truly effective first aid treatment to perform. On skin surfaces, soap and water may be used. Do not delay the cleansing process. The sooner done after exposure to Mace, the better the results. If the agent has gotten on the subject's clothing, the subject should be given the opportunity to shower and put on a set of clean jail garments.

There are certain situations that demand that the subject exposed to Mace be taken immediately to the local hospital emergency room for medical treatment that a *physician* deems warranted. These situations are:

1. Discharge of the CN weapon straight into the face or

eyes of the subject at close range (less than 2 feet)
2. Lengthy discharge of CN at any effective range into the face of a person already incapacitated
3. Discharge of a large amount of agent in a limited space such as cubicle, closed automobiles, or closet

Orthochlorobenzylidenemalononitrile, CS

The chemical formula is ClC$_6$H$_4$CHC) CN)$_2$. The following are important characteristics of CS:

Molecular weight	188.5
Melting point	93° to 95°C (199° to 302°F)
Boiling point	310° to 315°C (590° to 599°F)
Stability	Stable
Odor	Pepperlike
Not readily hydrolyzed	

CS is the official riot control agent of the United States Department of Defense. The agent is incorporated into civilian-type riot control and personal protection agents and devices such as Paralyzer®.

Extensive research is summarized in the following statement generated by the world-famous Edgewood Arsenal in Maryland (1967).

CS is the symbol identifying a riot control agent which has come into prominence in the last few years and is increasingly finding favor over the more familiar "tear gas" of the past. CS has sometimes been referred to as super-tear gas because of its more potent action. It is, however, an extremely safe material to use in spite of its potency. The Army made CS its standard riot control agent in 1959 and has practically replaced the previous CN tear gas in stockpiles. CS has been widely disseminated to Army and National Guard units and its ready availability through several commercial sources has placed it in the hands of many law enforcement agencies.

CS takes its name from the two scientists, B. B. Corson and R. W. Stoughton, who first prepared it in 1928. Its descriptive name in the language of the chemist is ortho-chlorobenzalmalononitrile which favors the use of the symbol. Contrary to its common name, it is not a gas but is a white, crystalline powder, similar in appearance to talcum powder. To get it to its intended target rapidly, it is dispersed as an aerosol cloud of finely divided particles. This dispersal is accomplished by blowers or bursting grenades or by burning a mixture of the powder and a fuel. Riot control hardware is designed to avoid mechanical or physical injury on the target, grenade and other dispersal devices being small and light (in one case made of rubber).

The effects of CS are impressive. CS produces immediate effects even in low concentrations. The irritating effects of the compound are felt immediately and the duration of effects is 5 to 10 minutes after the affected individual is removed to fresh air. During this time, affected persons are incapable of effective concerted action. The agent cloud causes severe burning sensation in the eyes with copious tears, coughing and difficulty in breathing with tightness of chest. The eyes close involuntarily, the nose runs, and moist skin stings.

Area decontamination is not required as CS has a short duration of effectiveness in the concentrations used in riot control operations. Personnel exposed to CS may shower as necessary. When individuals are affected by CS, they should move to fresh air, face the wind and should *not* rub their eyes. If, in handling CS dissemination devices, a person receives accidental gross contamination, he should remove clothing and flush his body with large amounts of water to remove most of the agent. If available, a 5% sodium bisulfite solution is helpful in removing the remainder of the agent.

To understand the small amount of agent required for effects, this can be related to quantities we are more familiar with. The effective concentration for the average person is 10 to 20 milligrams per cubic meter. Twenty milligrams is a quantity about one sixth the amount in an ordinary saccharin tablet. A cubic meter is about 35 cubic feet and it takes a man about 66 minutes to need that much air. This means that a man remaining in an effective cloud for 1 minute will breathe only one sixty-sixth of that one-sixth of a saccharin tablet, or about one four-hundredth of the tablet.

Munitions when utilized efficiently produce concentrations which generally do not greatly exceed the effective dose. However, since unforeseen circumstances may occur in which higher concentrations are entered by individuals, it is necessary to know what the effect would be; i.e., what is the safety factor? First, it can be stated that CS has never been implicated in any death in man despite repeated use. Second, it was certified for use only after elaborate safety tests had been performed.

The physicians and toxicologists who were charged with this safety testing approached their tasks in a manner analagous to the testing of a new experimental drug. First resort was to extensive use of small rodents in carefully designed and humane experiments. Here the toxicologist determined the effect on the animal and, by gradually increasing dosages, determined the safety ratio. The investigation then extended to a number of other larger animal species to give insight into the reaction of diverse types. Lastly, the higher animals, the primates, were tested to make closer analogy to man. In these experiments, animals of different sexes, ages, and weights were used to determine the effects of these differences. Animals were given brief exposures or repeated exposures to determine this effect. In addition to observing the apparent response of the animal, clinical and pathological measurements were made to determine if unseen changes were occurring. Lastly after combining and reviewing all these results from lower animals experiments, since there were no contrary indications of toxic effects, volunteer men were tested to determine their response to the experimental chemical. It is obvious that volunteers were not given a dose much higher than an effective dose. The toxic dose level for the experimental animals can be used to estimate the safety factor for men.

The results of this extensive testing attest to the safety of CS. The combined data for mice, rats, guinea pigs, rabbits, dogs, and monkeys were used as the lethal estimate for men, despite the fact that this value ignores the more resistant swine, goats, sheep and burros. On this basis, a 2600 safety factor is provided. This means at least 2600 times as much as it required to affect man would be required to be fatal. If the swine, goat, sheep, and burro data were included, the safety estimate would rise to 15,000. This indicates that it is extremely unlikely that in field use lethal concentrations could ever be present.

Even more confidence in safety of CS has been developed from further toxicological studies. For example, monkeys and goats, ill with pneumonia, were not adversely affected by high concentrations of CS. Also, rats and dogs exposed for 5 weeks to repeated doses of CS showed no significant effects as shown by gross pathological examinations. Repeated exposures did not seem to make the animals more sensitive. To evaluate effects on the eye, CS was dropped in rabbits eyes. Only a temporary conjunctivitis resulted with no corneal damage. Finally, the response of men over 50 years of age or having medical histories of allergies, hypertension, jaundice, or hepatitis did not differ from that of young, healthy volunteers.

In summary, CS has been subjected to testing of a type typical for a new drug or medicine. These results, coupled with extensive field use, show CS to be a highly effective riot control agent, fast-acting, psychologically feared, but with a safety factor that makes the probability extremely low that lasting effects or death will come from its use in riot situations.

Recapitulation for CS

Orthochlorobenzylidene malononitrile was adopted by the United States Army in 1960 as a new chemical warfare agent. It was given the classification CS for identification purposes. It is a very powerful irritant that has been a favorite weapon of the police in the United States and other countries during the last few years for the control and suppression of demonstrations, gatherings, and the like. The Army has also used great quantities of CS without scruple in Vietnam.

As an aerosal, it has a powerful irritant effect on the eyes and the upper respiratory organs. Within a few seconds, a severe conjunctivitis develops, accompanied by a burning sensation, great pain, and flow of tears. With the exception of the conjunctivitis, the effects last only 5 to 10 minutes. As a rule, the persons affected are again capable of action after 5 to 10 minutes; although occasionally certain aftereffects occur (a "tired feeling" in the eyes and sensitivity to light). The intensity of the conjunctivitis decreases after 25 to 30 minutes.

The effect on the respiratory passages contributes most to the incapacitation for combat and action. At first there is a burning feeling in the laryngeal cavity, later a painful burning in the chest and a feeling of constriction. In severe intoxications, fear also occurs, which intensifies the whole symptomatic picture and makes the affected person disinclined to breathe either in or out. In fresh air, the symptoms rapidly disappear.

Other symptoms of CS intoxication are copious nasal discharge and flow of saliva, as well as great irritation in the nose. Occasionally, nosebleed has occurred among those working with CS. Headache, nausea, and lethargy are nonspecific and do not occur in all cases. There is strong burning sensation on the skin of affected parts, which is greatly aggravated by moisture (sweat, tears, and so forth). The skin irritation remains for some hours even after washing. With longer exposure or high concentrations, erythemata and blisters develop.

Dosage of 0.005 mg of orthochlorobenzylidene malononitrile

per liter of air is unendurable for periods of exposure longer than 1 minute. A concentration of 0.01 mg/liter has been endured about 12 seconds, and 0.034 mg/liter from 6 to 9 seconds. The concentration leading to combat incapacity is given as 0.001 to 0.005 mg/liter. Lethal concentrations are hardly to be expected under combat conditions.

Orthochlorobenzylidene malononitrile is prepared from ortho-chlorobenzaldehyde and malonic acid nitrile. It is a white substance that dissolves well in gasoline, trichloromethane, and acetone but less well in alcohol, tetrachloromethane, and water. It melts at 95°C and boils, turning dark, and 310° to 315°C (that is 760 mm of mercury pressure).

Orthochlorobenzylidene malononitrile is relatively resistant to hydrolysis. In a mixture of 95 percent ethanol and 5 percent water, the hydrolytic half-life is about 95 minutes at 30°C and 40 minutes at 40°C. After 635 minutes at 30°C, 99 percent has been hydrolyzed. The rate of hydrolysis is reduced by hydrogen ions, while hydrolysis is accelerated by hydroxyl ions. Oxidizing agents attack the double bonds in the molecule, forming various oxidation products. For example, with hypochloride, an epoxide is formed.

Biomedical Studies

The results of exhaustive research on "riot control agents" (primarily CN) have been published in a special symposium (Kalman, 1971). Low concentrations of riot control agents cause eye discomfort, profuse tears, and mild conjunctivitis (mild irritation of the conjunctiva of the eye). *Injury to the cornea of the eye does not occur in concentrations used for police work.*

High concentrations of CN striking the eye may result in some temporary corneal damage. Tear gas (CN) cartridges that are too old have agent that does not vaporize adequately; the resulting small particles of solid agent strike the cornea and cause damage. If at all possible, riot control agents one year old should be used only with great caution and under conditions that preclude their striking the eye. Riot control agents two years old should be destroyed.

There is no specific antidote for riot control agents; none is needed. Whether it is CS or CN that has been used against a subject, the first step in treatment is the same: copious floods of clean water in the eyes to wash out the eyes, or flooding the skin with water to cleanse it. Topical anesthetics or eye ointments must be avoided; they retard healing and can aggravate the injury. "Temporary discomfort is preferable to permanent injury from a topical anesthetic" (Kalman, 1971).

Rare cases of contact dermatitis are reported after exposure to CN-containing Chemical Mace, primarily in persons previously sensitized to chloroacetophenone (CN), if contact with the skin persists for 3 or more minutes.

Individuals who are in occupations or activities that result in frequent exposures to CN (chloroacetophenone) should remember that CN can sensitize one to further exposures and that the probability of developing dermatitis with a subsequent minimal exposure is appreciable.

The overall conclusion of the civilian biomedical symposium on police riot control agents was a clear recognition that low concentrations of these chemicals, especially CS, are effective for the intended purpose. Excessive concentrations, overage formulations, and careless use may result in undesirable side effects, a situation that is true for any chemical.

As is true for any chemical introduced into man's environment, there must be a balancing of the desired effects against unavoidable but possible detriment. If the riot control agents are used properly, their obvious value for the purposes intended greatly overshadows the infrequent unwanted toxic reactions that have been recorded. Both agents CN and CS have wide margins of safety in use. From the biological standpoint, CS seems to be the riot control agent of choice.

Neither of the two riot control agents now in use has been shown to produce other than transitory effects. There are no theoretical considerations nor observed responses in man or other animals that would suggest a systemic or generalized action of any of these agents on the heart, brain, muscle, or other organ system.

Table 7-I
CHARACTERISTICS OF MILITARY RIOT CONTROL AGENT CS*

Characteristic	Burning Type	Powder Type
Composition	CS; potassium chlorate; thiourea; magnesium carbonate	Micropulverized CS; silica; aerogel
Odor	Pungent; pepperlike	Pungent; pepperlike
Persistency (in open)	Variable according to wind conditions	Variable according to wind conditions; greater with lack of wind or in wooded terrain
Minimum effective protection	Protective mask; field clothing	Protective mask; field clothing
Physiological action	Extreme burning sensation of the eyes; copious flow of tears; coughing, difficult breathing, and chest tightness; involuntary closing of eyes; stinging action on moist skin areas; sinus and nasal drip; nausea and vomiting on exposure to extreme concentrations (via ingestion)	Extreme burning sensation of the eyes; copious flow of tears; coughing, difficult breathing, and chest tightness; involuntary closing of eyes; stinging action on moist skin areas; sinus and nasal drip; nausea and vomiting on exposure to extreme concentrations (via ingestion)
Time required for maximum effort	Immediate	Immediate
First aid	Remove to uncontaminated area; face into wind; caution against rubbing eyes; keep affected persons well spaced; shower after several hours. Shower first with cool water for 3 to 5 minutes, then proceed with normal showering. For gross accidental contamination with CS particles, flush body with copious amounts of cool water, then use a 5% sodium bisulfite	Remove to uncontaminated area; face into wind; caution against rubbing eyes; keep affected persons well spaced; shower after several hours. Shower first with cool water for 3 to 5 minutes, then proceed with normal showering. For gross accidental contamination with CS particles, flush body with copious amounts of cool water, then use a 5% sodium bisulfite

Table 7-I

CHARACTERISTICS OF MILITARY RIOT CONTROL AGENT CS* *(Continued)*

Characteristic	Burning Type	Powder Type
	solution (except in and around eyes), and finally flush again with water. A 1% solution of sodium carbonate or sodium bicarbonate may be substituted for sodium bisulfite solution.	solution (except in and around eyes), and finally flush again with water. A 1% solution of sodium carbonate or sodium bicarbonate may be substituted for sodium bisulfite solution.
Type of munitions	Grenades, hand and rifle	Grenades, hand
Mechanically dispersable	No	Yes

*(Department of the Army, 1968)

Chapter 8

SPECIAL PROBLEMS WITH CHILDREN

CHILDREN PRESENT A SPECIAL PROBLEM with respect to poisoning. They are biologically immature and hence, in general, are more susceptible to the toxic action of a wide variety of chemicals. In addition, their comparatively small mass (light weight compared to adults) makes a given amount of a poison in effect a larger dose in terms of weight of the poison per unit of body weight. The inquisitive behavior of all children and their lack of experience makes every poison in their vicinity a real hazard to their health and welfare.

Poisoning Accidents to Children

The frequency of poisoning accidents during childhood has increased recently in all countries of the world that keep such statistics. A study covering twelve years involving some 356 infants and children who were treated for accidental poisoning showed that the incidence of such poisoning was highest in the second and third years of life. The incidence then fell off sharply by seven years of age. More than 95 percent of these poisonings happened in the home. Some of these were the result of an incorrect prescription given by a doctor for the child; these cases accounted for over 6 percent of the accidental poisonings. The most frequent kind of poisoning was from medicines, which accounted for 39 percent of the cases. Next in frequency were the ordinary household chemicals, which accounted for about 25 percent of the poisonings. Other toxic agents included insecticides, rat poisons, poisonous plants, gases, alcohol, and mercury. The majority of the poisonings were found to be due to carelessness on the part of parents. If there is to be a reasonable decrease in accidental child-hood poisonings, there must be cooperation, especially by parents, to keep children away from toxic materials. There is no possibility of training children to be mentally alert, not inquisitive, and have the level of judgment that adults are supposed to have (Reddemann and Amendt, 1968).

Of the accidental poisonings each year in the United States, approximately 500 cases occur in children who are five years old or younger (Done, 1968). In this group of children, poisoning by lead is the third most frequent cause of death. It is also the main cause of mental retardation. As many as 10 severe cases of lead poisoning are documented for every fatal case recorded.

For these reasons, it is essential that poisonous materials of all sorts be kept out of the reach of children. Law enforcement officers can render a useful community service by reminding citizens of the need to keep poisons away from curious young ones under all circumstances.

Child-Proof Containers

There has been a move to have potentially hazardous materials dispensed in "child-proof" containers. These containers are a mixed blessing. Their construction is such that they may inhibit the explorations of the average child for a time. However, such containers pose a severe hazard to adults who may have heart disease that requires the quick taking of a medication when an attack occurs; for persons with arthritis that prevents full effective use of joints, especially those in the hand; and for older and debilitated persons who just have a physical incapacity in carrying out effectively any demanding physical manipulation. There are no strong data to justify the universal use of such child-proof containers. There are clear justifications for urging that households in which children reside or visit should keep all potentially poisonous chemicals and chemical formulations in a *locked* cabinet with the key available only to the parents, in a secure place away from prying hands of little ones.

Hazards of Household Chemicals

As examples of the household chemicals that pose real threats to the health and welfare of children, consider the following. Let us start with the living room and the crayons that may be there for helping a child through a rainy day. These crayons may contain aniline dyes in amounts sufficient to cause poisoning if enough of the substance is swallowed by a child. Red-colored crayons in particular may have the toxic paranitraniline in them. In the master bedroom, the child may come in contact with depilatories containing soluble sulfide of barium as well as sodium or calcium thioglycollate. Moth balls may also be found there, as well as deodorant preparations. Many bedrooms may have some barbiturates about; these are sinister threats for children and adults unless used under carefully controlled and informed conditions. In the bathroom medicine cabinet are aspirin, other salicylate formulations, cathartics, and nitrites. As the child moves into the dining room, he may encounter copper sulfate and cyanide in the silver polish. In the kitchen, often in a cupboard under the sink, are such items as roach-killing powder, rat poison, lye, shoe dyes, and other dyes. When the child plays in the garage, possible exposure to kerosene, degreasing compounds, weed killers, and insecticides may result. Outdoors in the yard, fields, and woods, there are toadstools (poisonous mushrooms), Jimson weed, and an assortment of poisonous berries.

These are only a few of the toxic hazards that surround the growing child. The point of all this is that parents must be regularly exhorted to protect their own children from these chemical hazards. It is unrealistic to assume or demand that a government office, a manufacturer, or "the schools" should be responsible for such protection. Law enforcement personnel can carry out a valuable teaching function by letting the public know, in a helpful and effective manner, that these hazards exist and how children can be protected from everyday poisonous substances in the home.

Moth Crystals and Balls

Moth repellant compounds are often found about the home. There is some indication that vacation homes occupied for only part of the year may have these materials about more frequently than the year-round home. The moth crystals (snow, cakes, flakes) are made up of the chemical paradichlorobenzene. It is relatively nontoxic, although exposure for a long period of time can cause cataracts and damage to the liver. Moth balls are usually made up of the chemical naphthalene. A 2 gm amount (1/14th ounce) ingested is known to have caused death in a child. The average fatal dose is more than that. Naphthalene is readily soluble in oils. Baby oil dissolves it and facilitates the absorption of the chemical through the skin.

Iron Poisoning

Acute poisoning by iron is among the common forms of fatal childhood poisoning in the United States. It usually results from the child's swallowing ferrous sulfate tablets prescribed for a pregnant woman in the household, most probably the child's mother (Public Health Service, 1973). Swallowing of 10 to 15 five-grain tablets has proven fatal to children.

Poisoning symptoms develop in 30 to 90 minutes; they include signs of shock, coma, acidosis, vomiting, diarrhea, and melena (black, tarry feces). Untreated, the child may seem to improve, but by 10 to 14 hours after the intake of poison, further acidosis, coma, bleeding, and irreversible shock occur; the child expires. The biological mechanism of action is obscure. Autopsy results are not specific.

These cases demand immediate medical attention to prevent death. The drug deferoxamine, to be used only under close medical supervision, has shown promise of significantly decreasing deaths from acute iron poisoning.

Methodology in Lead Poisoning

Lead poisoning is common in many groups of urban children. The two common routes of lead entry into the body are through the lungs and by way of the digestive system (Berman, 1966). Lead poisoning in children usually results from the swallowing of lead. Industrial poisonings by lead are usually caused by inhalation of lead fumes or dusts.

Organic lead compounds pass through intact human skin with ease. Once lead gets into the body, it is distributed to all organs of the body. At first the liver and kidneys show the highest amounts of lead. Soon the lead moves from those organs and is deposited in bone, where it is effectively in dead storage. Lead leaves the body in feces, urine, and sweat.

Lead in the urine reveals the amount of lead absorbed by the body. Lead values in blood are meaningless except in acute poisoning cases. In chronic cases of lead poisoning, blood levels reveal little. Suggested guidelines for interpreting blood levels of lead are shown in Table 8-I.

Table 8-I
BLOOD LEVELS OF LEAD

$\mu g/100\ ml$	Interpretation
0-21	Negative
21-60	Increased lead exposure
above 60	Dangerous

For demonstrating lead in body fluids, body organs, or other materials that might contain lead, atomic absorption flame spectrophotometry is the method of choice because of its sensitivity, specificity, and ease of execution.

In a study of 1645 cases of child poisonings, it was found that 35 percent were caused by medicines, 25 percent were caused by corrosives, 22 percent were attributed to lead paint or plaster, and the balance were caused by household chemicals. Of the children who showed brain damage from lead poisoning, 27 percent died.

A Form of Child Abuse

Medical experts in Great Britain have called attention to the need to look at each case of child poisoning as a potential form of child cruelty or abuse *(Rocky Mountain News,* 1976) .

In our pill-popping society, there is evidence that cases of adults giving children drugs of various forms as a type of abuse or maltreatment is no longer a remote consideration. The British experts urged emergency room personnel as well as other appropriate medical and paramedical workers to become suspicious when children are brought to their care showing unexplained bizarre signs of poisoning. Cases of repeated episodes of this sort are particularly to be suspected. Among the signs that were fairly common in the British experience were difficulty in breathing and drowsiness.

There have been reported in the United States no similar cases. It may be that poisoning as a form of child abuse is culturally limited, or it might be that the present methodology of handling child poisoning cases in the United States has not lent itself to uncovering cases of frank abuse.

In Great Britain, the incidence of child abuse is not insignificant; over 73,000 cases are known to have been handled in 1974 in England. Medical opinion in England leans toward blaming much of cruelty to children on "stresses that plague modern society." Poisoning as a form of child abuse is said to derive from the parent's own psychiatric problems. According to British view, the deliberate poisoning of a child permits parents to get away from their personal mental, physical, or marital troubles. One psychiatric opinion in England is that poisoning of a child as a form of abuse may be a gesture of suicide somehow related to poisoning oneself. Several cases have been reported by the British medical experts.

> A two-year-old female child was given diabetes control pills regularly by the diabetic father for more than six months. The child died. Toxicologists might wish to urge pathologists to keep such a possibility in mind in the event of unexplainable deaths in young children.

> For three years, the mother of a seven-year-old male had fed the child potent sleeping pills on a steady basis. The mother was a depressed, suicidal sort. When confronted with her abusing behavior, she agreed to psychiatric treatment.

> A six-year-old male, the third child of a twenty-one-year-old mother, was truly an unwanted child. The mother had developed multiple sclerosis. She had fed barbiturates to the child for a period of four years. The boy was turned over to a care center; the woman was given psychiatric treatment.

Strange unaccountable behavior in children or child deaths that seem to defy a clear cause might well be looked at as possible cases of chronic poisoning, usually with some chemical that one of the parents has reasonably ready access to.

Acrodynia

Acrodynia is a reddening and itching of the hands and feet. This condition is associated particularly with what is called the *pink disease,* which is a form of mercury poisoning. Many times a law enforcement officer may be called to a home where a child shows general signs and symptoms of poisoning that may be related to excessive intake of mercury.

> An eight-year-old-girl had experienced about 4 weeks of irritability, sweating, generalized pain, and a reddish rash that eventually faded but was followed by an itchy, blistery eruption of the hands and feet. She was admitted to a hospital, where she showed signs of distress. She lay in the fetal position with her limbs rigidly bent. She sweated profusely despite the fact that her body temperature was normal. She showed no particular pain as a result of bright lights. Chemical analysis of her blood serum and urine showed elevated amounts of mercury. She was immediately treated with injections of dimercaprol into muscle. Because there seemed to be no obvious source of mercury poisoning, her parents and five sisters were all given urine mercury tests. They all showed elevated levels of mercury in the urine; none showed signs and symptoms of mercury poisoning. Careful examination of the house and questioning of the family revealed that the source of mercury was a can of liquid mercury taken from school by one of the children of the family and with which all the children in this particular family played each day (Alexander and Rosario, 1971).

Acrodynia shows a number of symptoms. Fortunately, the disease is not common, but it is not entirely absent from human populations. The proper diagnosis can be made only if a clearly drawn clinical picture is available.

A recent case involved a girl seven years old who had acrodynia complicated by rectal prolapse (the falling down of the rectum through the anus so that it protrudes outside the body), attacks of severe difficulty in breathing, widespread ulcers, spontaneous breakages of bones, and a variety of secondary infections. A police officer investigating such a case might well conclude that child abuse or child neglect was the causative agent. However, more complete information about all the conditions surrounding this case indicated clearly that mercury from a defective dental filling was the agent causing the signs and symptoms exhibited by this girl (Schoene et al., 1970).

Treatment

An important point in all these considerations of metal poisoning in children is the fact that these various kinds of metal poisoning can be successfully treated by competent medical teams if adequate information is gathered as part of the case history of any child brought for medical attention because of suspected metal poisoning. It is further extremely important that the child be brought to medical attention before permanent or irreversible damage results to such organs as the brain, liver, or kidneys. Metal poisoning is so devastating when left untreated that all members of the community must be particularly alert to the possibility of such a plague affecting children in their surroundings.

The general treatment of any of the nervous system pathologies resulting from toxic metals or drugs, for that matter, is primarily removal from the source of poisoning. After that, the victim must be given appropriate symptomatic treatment.

Arsenic damage to the nervous system has been reported after acute and chronic poisonings. The mechanism of action is not clear, but treatment with dimercaprol is indicated for at least 10 days. In cases of severe arsenic poisoning in children, the disability the child experiences is a long one; permanent crippling is almost universal in the very severe cases.

Lead damage to the nervous system is much more common in adults than it is in children. Dimercaprol has no value in treating lead poisoning. However, there are two other drugs, calcium disodium EDTA and penicillamine, known to be effective in the treatment of lead poisoning.

Mercury damage to the nervous system commonly occurs after the swallowing of some household medicine or other chemical that contains mercury. For adequate treatment, dimercaprol must be given in large doses as soon as possible after the mercury exposure. It is highly effective in treating this poison, and if the treatment is initiated soon enough and vigorously enough, there should be no permanent damage. The devastation that mercury poisoning has brought to many societies around the world has been graphically described by D'Itri and D'Itri (1977, 1978). Children and unborn babies are particularly susceptible to the poisonous action of mercury.

Thallium damage to the nervous system follows the accidental swallowing of rodenticides or insecticides. Adults may be exposed to thallium in industry during the manufacture of sulfuric acid from iron pyrite (fool's gold). There is no specific treatment for thallium poisoning.

How to Prevent Childhood Poisoning?

The attack on the problem of accidental poisoning is a community responsibility. It involves the close collaboration between the poison control center, local health department, media of communications, schools, doctors, pharmacists, public health nurses, social workers, and various families in the communities. Poison control centers are equipped to supply critical information about the types of poisonings occurring, to whom they occur, and how frequently they are reported. The doctor, of course, treats poisoned patients. He should also be aware of the risks of repetition and should question the child's parents, arranging for them to be visited by a public health worker if necessary. The physician should also see that his prescriptions are properly and adequately labeled.

The pharmacist, in turn, must insist on safe precautions. He must spread the necessary information about the safe handling of prescription drugs. He truly is in a key position to help prevent many cases of childhood poisoning. Nurses and social workers have an educational role in the prevention of childhood poisonings. In the United States, the mass media have been used for public educational programs designed to create an awareness of the dangers of accidental poisoning. Preschool children are at the greatest risk from these toxic exposures. Educational programs for a child of preschool age should be informational rather than preventive. Using the school children as a way to reach the parents and preschool siblings is an effective route. Some community programs have been concerned with specific problems of poisoning, particularly lead poisoning from paint in old houses. Because of the widespread lead poisoning hazard and because of the devastating permanent effects that chronic lead poisoning may have, such emphasis is clearly warranted.

Container Design

Safety packaging has helped to reduce poisoning from prescription medicines. There is a growing use of child-resistant containers, but the use of these is not universally acclaimed. There is some evidence attempting to show that the rate of poisoning from substances packed in child-resistant containers is lower than the general average, and two-thirds of the cases that did occur were due to a misuse of the child-resistant containers. Safe packaging is not by any means a substitute for parental responsibility and vigilance, child guidance, or safe storage principles. The use of child-resistant containers for medicines for the elderly or for those afflicted with arthritis or other crippling diseases may be strongly opposed because of the hazard they present to individuals who do not have full use of their hands and fingers (Scherz, 1970).

What to Do When Poison Strikes

When poisoning is suspected, treatment should start immediately; someone should be sent to get a physician but first aid must begin as quickly as possible. Suppose you are alone and have no one near at hand to send for medical help. For the following poisons, you can begin immediately the proper first aid care: inhaled poisons, skin contamination, contamination of the eye, poisons that are injected, and chemical burns.

Ingested Poisons

Always call a physician first and immediately. If the physician gives instructions by phone, carry them out; if he directs that you do nothing until he or an ambulance arrives, follow his directions rigidly. Swallowed petroleum products must not be treated by inducing vomiting. Among these poisons are kerosene, lighter fluid, and gasoline. Vomiting can cause more damage than good.

Similarly, if corrosive poisons have been swallowed, vomiting must not be induced. There are two general types of corrosive poisons—acids and alkalies. The following acids are most commonly found around the home and in the general surroundings of the average citizen: hydrochloric acid; sulfuric acid, which is a component of metal cleaners and polishes; glacial (very strong) acetic acid; hydrofluoric acid; and antirust compounds. For these poisons, milk should be given; copious amounts of water are also helpful; 1 teaspoon of milk of magnesia in a cup of water is also a usual first aid measure.

Common poisonous alkalies include paintbrush cleaners, metal cleaners, ammonia water, window cleaners, washing soda (sodium carbonate), and some dishwashing and laundry compounds. First aid treatment depends on administration by mouth of milk, fruit juice, or vinegar.

For noncorrosive poisons that are swallowed such as aspirin or barbiturates, vomiting should be induced. Syrup of ipecac may be given; it should safely induce vomiting. Another useful emetic (vomiting-inducing agent) is made of 2 tablespoons of ordinary table salt in a glass of *warm* water. A finger or a spoon (bowl end) can be pushed to the back of the victim's throat and then gently pressed forward; vomiting usually results from that manipulation. When the victim begins to vomit, turn him face down and be sure that the hips are elevated so that none of the vomited material (vomitus) runs into the lungs.

Injected Poisons

These poisons are venoms introduced into the body by snakebite, scorpion bite, or the bite of some other poisonous animal. The victim should be made to lie down. A tourniquet should be tied around the affected extremity between the point of injection and the heart. An ice pack should be applied to the site of the injection. DO NOT ALLOW THE VICTIM TO WALK. Have him carried to a physician or to a hospital. Alcohol in any form must not be permitted for the victim; it only makes the toxic situation worse.

Inhaled Poisons

Inhaled poisons include carbon monoxide found in many gas fumes, carbon tetrachloride as a component of cleaning fluids as well as fire-extinguisher fluids and a variety of solvents, and ammonia. The victim must be removed immediately to fresh air. DO NOT PERMIT HIM TO WALK. Loosen his clothing so that breathing is in no way restricted. If breathing has stopped or is spasmodic, administer artificial respiration; mouth-to-mouth procedure is preferred. Keep the victim warm. The victim must not be permitted to be physically active. Alcohol in any form must be avoided; it makes the poisoning situation worse.

Contamination of the Skin

Various chemicals such as pesticides or aniline dyes are the common skin contaminants of concern. Remove the victim from source of contamination. Begin washing the skin thoroughly with copious amounts of water; a shower, faucet, hose, or even a shallow rapidly running stream or creek can be used as the water source. Simultaneously with the washing process, the clothing of the victim must be removed and discarded. Medical help must be summoned.

Contamination of the Eye

Ammonia and various other alkalies and acids are the chief offenders here. Riot control agents also get into the eye at times. The eyelids should be held open and the eye should be flushed with a *gentle,* copious stream of water. Ideally, the water should be about body temperature, neither hot nor cold. The flushing of the eye should be kept up until medical help arrives. SPEED of first aid treatment is crucial. UNDER NO CIRCUMSTANCES SHOULD CHEMICALS OF ANY SORT BE APPLIED TO THE EYE as part of the first aid treatment of eye contamination.

Chemical Burns

Acids and alkalies are the usual agents that cause chemical burns. The affected part of the body should be flooded with water and the process continued until it is reasonably certain that all the contaminant has been washed away. Then a clean cloth should be applied lightly to the burned area. Keep the victim lying down and keep him warm. Give no kind of medication as part of the first aid treatment. Apply *no* medication to the burned part; this warning applies especially to the smearing of greasy materials over the burn.

Table 8-II

TOXIC THREATS TO CHILDREN

Kitchen	*Bathroom*
Polishes and waxes (kerosene, oils, caustics, turpentine, oxalic acid)	Iron compounds, mercurial compounds, atropine eye drops, iodine, belladonna preparations
Detergents (strong alkaline solutions)	Hair dyes, tints (ammonium hydroxide, sodium hypachlorite solution, metallic dyes)
Dry cleaning fluids (carbon tetrachloride, kerosene, petroleum distillates)	Shampoos (denatured alcohol, sodium hexametaphosphate)
Insecticides (DDT, chlordane, benzene hexachloride)	Rubbing alcohol, depilatories (calcium thioglycolate, sulfides)
Ammonia solutions, moth balls, moth flakes (naphthalene)	Suntan lotions (denatured alcohol)
Rat poisons (phosphorus)	Tranquilizing drugs
	Digitalis (used for some types of heart disease)
Garage	
Paints, putty, varnishes (arsenic, cadmium, lead)	Aspirin
Paint removers (benzene, kerosene, carbon tetrachloride)	Boric acid
Paintbrush cleaners (acetone, turpentine, naphtha)	
Antifreeze (alcohols, ethylene glycol)	*Bedroom*
Antirust products (sodium nitrite, hydrofluoric acid)	Crayons (aniline dyes)
	Paint on crib (lead)
Fire-extinguishing fluids (carbon tetrachloride)	Lead toys
	Nail preparations (organic solvents)
Metal cleaners (acids and alkalies)	Cuticle removers (alkalies)
Drainpipe cleaner (lye)	Sleeping pills (barbiturates)
Fumes from engine (carbon monoxide)	

Some Characteristics of Childhood Poisonings

There is strong evidence that a child who has survived a poisoning experience once is more prone to additional episodes. The once-poisoned child is at a greater risk of suffering another poisoning than is the general population of its peers (Harris, 1966).

Furthermore, accidental poisonings in children are not uncommon. Poisoning of children happens at all economic and social levels; the poorer classes or the lower social classes do not show an elevated rate of such poisonings. The most probable victim is a two-year-old boy. There are certain families and certain individual children who seem to be poison prone. Families that have experienced one poisoning of a member show an elevated probability of going through further poisonings.

Children who are known to have been poisoned share in common the following characteristics: they are daredevils, highstrung, impulsive, overly active, and masculine. Females who belong to a once-poisoned group of children are twice as frequently described by their mothers as exhibiting boyish traits than are girls from nonpoisoned children. Poisoned children as a group are more likely to be among those who rebel against discipline (Table 8-II).

Chapter 9

INORGANIC AND METALLIC POISONS

THE USE OF INORGANIC SUBSTANCES, especially metals, for poisoning human beings was recognized at the dawn of written history. Accidental or occupational poisoning with metals was known as soon as man began to mine metallic elements as a regular occupation.

Hand in hand with the poisoning of human beings by inorganic and metallic elements has been the search for antidotes. The intensity of the search for antidotes against metallic and inorganic poisons has oscillated with the frequency of use of the poisons in question. When poisons were used politically and socially to get rid of undesirable individuals, the search for antidotes was vigorous. Later, when occupational diseases could be demonstrated as being associated with various inorganic chemicals and metallic poisons, a resurgence of vigorous research on possible antidotes occurred (Ulmer, 1973). "The quest for antidotes has a long history which early paralleled the popularity of poisons as instruments of assassination, and more recently, the advent of powerful drugs, the prevalence of opportunities for industrial exposure, and the impetus provided by an increased understanding of toxicologic mechanisms" (Done, 1961).

Antidotes

Antidotes are chemicals or chemical combinations that are useful in destroying the effect of a poison on a human being; they may be either mechanical or chemical in their action. Among the mechanical antidotes are cathartics, which serve to stimulate the intestine and thus to empty out as completely as possible the intestine and carry away any poisons that may have passed that far

down in the digestive tract. Emetics are also used. These medicines have the unique capacity of causing the individual to vomit
up any material that may be in the stomach. Again, this action
helps to get rid of poison still in the digestive tract but not yet
absorbed into the body. Finally, there are mechanically acting
demulcents. A demulcent is a slimy, mucilaginous fluid that alleviates irritation of the gut and soothes any inflammation that may
have resulted from the action of the poison on the mucous membranes lining the intestinal tract.

Chemical antidotes of various sorts, soaps, milk, tannins, and
oxidation and reducing substances, have been used alone or in
combination to ward off the effects of poisons. Most of the antidotes available are nonspecific and consequently have restricted
use. The so-called universal antidotes sometimes found in first aid
packages are nonspecific and of limited value.

On the other hand, there are a few specific antidotes now available for use against individual toxic agents. These antidotes are
usually complex chemicals that have synthesized by chemists
in a tailor-made fashion to work against a specific chemical whose
biochemical action in the human body is known.

An ideal antidote should first stop the destructive action of the
poison that is affecting the victim. Secondly, this ideal antidote
should undo the harm caused to the body by restoring the body
chemistry to a normal range.

The production of an ideal antidote requires a deep understanding of the basic physiology of the cell. We still have only a
relatively superficial knowledge of the functions of the cytoplasm
of the cell, despite the enormous advances made over the last
quarter of a century in cell physiology and biochemistry.

Chelating Agents

For the treatment of metal poisoning, there is now available a
group of compounds called chelating agents. These are organic
molecules that can form complexes with polyvalent metallic ions;
this complexing renders the metal causing the toxic action not
available to take part in its usual chemical reactions. There are
numerous substances with the potential for chelating materials,

although the number of such agents studied from the point of view of use as antidotes is limited. Nevertheless, as a result of intensive biomedical research on specific poisons, much of it as a direct offshoot of the requirements of chemical warfare defense, there are now available for physicians a number of chelating agents that are highly effective in treating metallic poisonings.

General Treatment of Poisoning

In the treatment of any kind of poisoning incident, the general approach to handling the situation involves essentially three procedures:

1. General nonspecific measures include the administration of emetics, cathartics, or diluents. This latter approach to treatment is sometimes quite effective. Many kinds of corrosive materials can be treated by the ingestion of milk, which dilutes the corrosive substance and thus prevents further damage to the stomach or intestine.
2. Physiological and pharmacological antagonists may be administered to the poisoned victim.
3. Direct chemical neutralization and detoxication of the poisonous agent may be possible.

At the present time, the first approach is most widely used in emergency and, indeed, in the long-term treatment of poisons.

British Anti-Lewisite, BAL

An example of a specific antidote for metallic poisons is seen in the development of British anti-lewisite, the chemical known as dimercaprol. Originally, this poison antidote was developed by British biochemists as a response to the arsenic-containing war gas called *lewisite* that the Germans proposed to use on the World War I battlefields. A British biochemist thoroughly studied the action of such arsenic-containing poisons as they behave in the human body. When this fundamental information on the action of arsenic-containing poisons was available, there was a tailor-made chemical that could counteract and prevent the action of such arsenic-containing compounds.

BAL was first used for counteracting the effects of arsenical-containing war gases. We now find that it is an effective antidote for several metallic poisons (Edds, 1950).

Dimercaprol, or British anti-lewisite, is chemically known as 2,3-dimercaptol propanol. Its chemical structure follows.

H H H
| | |
H-C-C-C-OH
| | |
S S H
H H
BAL

The molecular weight of BAL is 124.2. Its specific gravity is 1.21. The substance is an oily colorless liquid that has a strong odor of garlic. It is soluble in water up to about 6% (weight/volume) and oxidizes readily. It can be obtained as a preparation for use in the emergency treatment of poisonings in the form of 10% dimercaprol plus 20% benzyl benzoate in peanut oil. The preparation is injected into the muscles of an individual who has been subjected to certain metallic poisons.

Injury by Metals

The poisoning of individuals from lead, mercury, arsenic, thallium, cadmium, iron, gold, and copper gives a pattern of toxicity that is variable but reveals several organs as being damaged. These metallic poisons do not injure a single organ but do, in fact, cause damage to several organs.

In order for a physician or pathologist to make an accurate diagnosis of metal poisoning, it is important that chemical tests identify the heavy metal in blood, urine, fingernails, and possibly in the hair.* In addition, environmental objects such as food,

---

*There is serious question whether trace-element analysis of human hair from any part of the body in either sex gives reliable results with respect to levels of concentration of a given element. Laboratory wash treatments and other preparatory manipulations of human hair samples before analysis do little to erase the questionable nature of the analytical data. Data on trace elements in the human body obtained from analysis of hair samples cannot at the present time be accepted as meaningful and should not form a basis for expert testimony in court (Hilderbrand and White, 1974).

paint, air, water, and other materials should also be subjected to chemical tests to demonstrate the presence of suspected metals.

There are special drugs that can be used in the treatment of metal poisonings, among them are calcium disodium edetate, dimercaprol, D-penicillamine, and deferoxamine. These drugs are important and can be lifesaving in heavy metal poisonings. However, these *chelating agents,* as they are called, are used differently from one metal to another. None of these chelating agents is a universal antidote for metal poisonings.

Consequently, it is critical that there be an accurate chemical identification of the heavy metal causing the poisoning of a given person if proper therapy or treatment is to be initiated. The essential aspect of identifying chemically the environmental source of a victim's exposure to poison should be obvious if recurrence of the exposure to this poison is to be circumvented. Chemical analysis of body tissues and body fluids will reveal the severity of the poisoning, which will determine the specific kind of treatment the victim will undergo. For example, an important principal of chelation treatment is the rule that an adequate molar excess of chelating agent above the toxic heavy metal must be provided. If insufficient chelating agent is used, the poisoning action of the metal may be intensified. Thus, fairly accurate information should be available to the physician to insure that an excess of the treatment drug be given to the patient (Chisolm, 1970).

Trace Metals and the Brain

A number of trace metals are found in brain tissue. When a specific metal is found in excess amounts as a result of poisoning, it acts as a cell poison. It is possible that the specific metal acts directly on a certain important enzyme system in the cell. Manganese, for example, seems to be an essential metal in human nutrition. In the brain, there is more manganese in the occipital lobe, which is at the back of the brain, than in other parts of the brain. Experiments with animals deficient in manganese show that the animals have a lower threshold for epilepticlike seizures than do animals with normal manganese levels. Miners who work in the manganese industry develop parkinsonian conditions.

Zinc is an interesting metal because it is required in very small amounts for normal functioning of the body. However, mild zinc deficiencies can result in a number of diseases. The zinc content of the hair is said to be a useful guide for revealing zinc deficiency in man.

Mercury exerts its activity by poisoning enzymes that are necessary for the orderly functioning of the human body. Inorganic mercury poisoning is primarily a hazard of industry (Cumont, 1972). Historically, inorganic mercury was used by some poisoners with homicidal intent. Poisoning from organic mercury occurs in industry or may result from accidental swallowing of an organic mercury compound.

Copper is, under normal conditions, taken into the body in the amount of 2 to 5 mg each day. Most of that intake leaves the body in the feces. Virtually every tissue and body fluid in the human organism contains copper. Of special importance is the copper found in a number of proteins essential to the normal functioning of the body. However, copper itself is poisonous to many enzyme systems. There is a condition known as *Wilson's disease* that is characterized by the deposition of copper in many tissues of the body, especially in the brain and in the liver. One suggestion about the origin of this disease is that as a result of a failure in the manufacture of ceruloplasmin, the copper that normally would go into that copper-containing protein is deposited where it can cause harm. There are certain chelating agents that are useful in removing the excess copper from the body. The disease itself is associated with mental abnormalities (Cumings, 1967).

Arsenic Poisoning

The water-soluble salts of the metal arsenic are absorbed through the mucous membranes of the body. If arsenic is made into certain medical ointments, it can be absorbed through the skin. Arsenic is carried by the blood from the point of absorption to where it is deposited in specific tissues. Biochemical evidence at the present time indicates that arsenic combines with sulfur in the various cells of the body. The chief storage locations for arsenic in the human body are the liver, kidneys, walls of the digestive tract, spleen, and lungs.

Relatively large amounts of arsenic at times are found in the hair or nails. "Deposition in the hair starts within two weeks after administration and arsenic stays fixed at this state for years. It is also deposited in bone and retained there for long periods" (Morrell, 1978).

If arsenic is administered by a vein, a large amount is eliminated from the body by the kidneys. The kidneys begin to excrete arsenic between 2 and 8 hours after the arsenic enters the body. Nevertheless, it may require as much as 10 days for the total elimination of arsenic given in a single dose. If several doses are given in succession, the time for complete elimination may be as much as 70 days. Because arsenic is so slowly eliminated, it can produce a cumulative poisoning action on the body.

There are two types of arsenic poisoning: acute and chronic. Acute poisoning usually occurs after swallowing an inorganic form of arsenic. About 100 mg taken by mouth is a poisonous dose, the arsenic in the form of powdered arsenic trioxide.

How soon do signs and symptoms of acute poisoning develop? It depends on how fast the arsenic is absorbed by the body. There are cases in which arsenic was swallowed along with a meal; the signs and symptoms of poisoning did not occur until 12 hours after the poison was swallowed. Usually within an hour after swallowing arsenic there is recognizable discomfort in the digestive tract. The individual feels a tightening of the throat and difficulty in swallowing. Very soon after this, agonizing pain in the stomach begins. The slightest pressure over the stomach makes the pain intolerable. The individual vomits vigorously—a form of vomiting known as projectile vomiting. The vomited material consists at first of a milky watery fluid, which later becomes slimy and tinged with a greenish color with bloody streaks.

Diarrhea is violent. Very soon, the material passed has a rice water appearance. Eventually, blood is mixed with the diarrheal fluid. Urine is suppressed; but urine that is produced may have large amounts of albumin and blood. The kidneys shut down and do not produce any more urine. The victim complains of cramps in the muscles. The massive loss of fluid in vomiting and in diarrhea brings on a severe thirst.

Because of the upset of the fluid balance and electrolytes in the body fluids, the individual begins to show the signs and symptoms of shock. The skin is cold to the touch, damp, and pale. The pulse has a high rate but is weak. The blood pressure is decreased, and respiration is inhibited. Coma and death follow shortly thereafter. Near death, the individual may experience anoxia, which brings on convulsions. There are cases of severe arsenic poisoning in which death occurred within 60 minutes. Ordinarily, the period between ingestion of an acute dose of arsenic and death is about 24 hours.

Chronic arsenic poisoning is caused by the successive administration of, or exposure to, nontoxic amounts of arsenic. The successive doses from whatever source build up to toxic levels. The appearance of chronic poisoning with arsenic is truly insidious. First of all, the patient complains of being weak. There is a loss of appetite. Now and then, certain patients become sick and vomit. Diarrhea may occur, but in some cases the individual is constipated. As the toxic levels are increased, the signs and symptoms observed become more like what is expected in cases of acute arsenic poisoning. The chronically poisoned individual may show inflammation of the upper respiratory passages. There may be sneezing, hoarseness, and coughing, excessive salivation is reported, and inflammation around the mouth is also observed. In the chronically poisoned individual exposed to arsenic, dermatitis is often observed. There is an interesting color change or increase in pigmentation of the skin, which is given the name of *arsenic melanosis;* it is seen on the neck, around the eyes, around the nipples, and in the armpits. The skin may become scaly and sluff off.

Internal organs such as the liver swell up. The kidneys are damaged. Fluid accumulates in the eyelids, the face, and around the ankles. Hair and nails frequently fall out. If chronic arsenic poisoning continues, the nervous system is harmed. *"Arsenical encephalopathy* is the term used to designate the apathetic idiotic condition which results from long and severe exposure" (Morrell, 1978).

There are other signs of chronic arsenic poisoning, including inflammation of the outlying nerves of the body. This results in paralysis of the extremities. The legs seem to be more severely harmed than the arms. The bone marrow is also damaged. The most common first indications of chronic arsenic poisoning include diarrhea, pigmentation of the skin, hyperkeratosis, and circumscribed edema, especially of the lower eyelids and around the ankles. One interesting sign that should arouse suspicion is the garlic odor to the breath or the perspiration.

A number of reliable methods for identifying arsenic are available and are published in virtually all analytical chemistry books. Modern laboratories in which the atomic absorption spectrophotometer is used find this method much less cumbersome than the older methods. The development of an arsine generator makes the atomic absorption method routine. Modern analytical techniques result in reproducible and reliable results for arsenic in biological materials.

Action of Arsenic as a Poison

Arsenic has been known for centuries as a particularly potent poison when used against the human body. Arsenic attacks important sulfur-containing chemicals in the protoplasm of all the cells in the human body. If experimental animals are given certain chemicals that contain high amounts of sulfur, these animals then are resistant to the poisoning action of arsenic. There are other metals such as bismuth and mercury that have actions on the human body similar to that of arsenic.

There seems to be no question that the poisonous effect of arsenic results from its capacity to combine with and keep out of chemical reaction sulfur-containing chemicals in various body tissues. These sulfur-containing chemicals are important in the use of oxygen by these tissues. Moreover, this harmful effect can be delayed or partly reversed by giving the human subject chemicals that contain high amounts of sulfur in the proper combination.

The antidotal action of British anti-lewisite results from the capacity of the British anti-lewisite to unite with the poisonous metal and form stable chemical compounds with the poison, thus preventing it from reaching the vital sulfur-containing chemicals involved in respiration of the tissues of the body. The interesting point is that the attraction of BAL for arsenic is so great that it can remove arsenic that already has partly damaged some of the sulfur-containing chemicals in the cell. In other words, BAL, because of its strong attraction for arsenic (and metals having similar actions), can reverse the toxic effect by removing the arsenic from the important tissue chemicals.

Arsenic may be a factor in the production of cancer of the skin. There is no valid reason for assuming that arsenic causes other kinds of cancer (Foreman, 1962).

Treatment with BAL

Ordinarily, individuals who are poisoned with arsenic fall into two categories—those individuals who have severe complications and those individuals who have mild complications. For severely poisoned individuals, a dose of BAL is given immediately in the amount of 3 mg of BAL for every kg of body weight. It must be remembered that the usual drug preparation of BAL has 10% BAL in solution in oil, or approximately 100 mg/ml of oil solution. On the first 2 days after severe poisoning, the subject is given six injections of the calculated dose, one every 4 hours. On the third day, four injections at 6-hour intervals are given. Over the next 10 days, two injections of the calculated dose are given each day.

For individuals who have milder complications, the dose is approximately 2.5 mg of BAL per kg of body weight. During the first 2 days, four injections are given at 6-hour intervals. On the third day, two injections are given. Thereafter, one or two injections are given each day for about 10 days or until complete recovery is observed.* The excretion of arsenic in the urine is monitored chemically in order to get a measure of the effectiveness of elimination of the poison.

The National Research Council of the United States (1977), an

---

*Chronic arsenic poisoning has been documented in persons who have been found to abuse (mostly unknowingly) arsenic-containing tonics (Leslie and Smith, 1978). The symptoms are mild, but tissue arsenic levels are high compared to those found in acute nonfatal arsenic poisonings. The study supports the view that long-term intake by mouth of arsenic leads to tolerance.

arm of the National Academy of Sciences, has published an excellent review of arsenic as an environmental pollutant. In order to cover the subject adequately, the monograph includes a large amount of toxicological information on arsenic that is of interest to the law enforcement community. The following information is included: arsenic chemistry, distribution, metabolism, and effects on plants, animals, and man. A valuable set of appendices include tables on the normal arsenic content of plants, plant products, and animals (Table 9-I) in addition to a digest of analytical methods for ascertaining the amounts of arsenic in unknown

Table 9-I

NORMAL RANGE OF ARSENIC CONTENT OF HUMAN BODIES*

Tissue	Arsenic concentration, ppm (fresh wt)	Tissue	Arsenic concentration, ppm (fresh wt)
Hair	0.3-1.75	Intestine	0.07
Distal	0.79	Spleen	0.08-0.13
Proximal	0.03-1.92		0.001-0.132†
	<3.0	Bone	0.16-0.50
Brain	0.997	Calvarium	59-61 (in ash)
	0.001-1.14†	Rib	20-27 (in ash)
Teeth	0.003-0.635	Nail	1.70
Thyroid	0.06-0.635		0.04-0.11
	0.001-0.314†		0.02-2.90†
	0.003-0.332†	Blood	0.01-0.59
Lung	0.08-0.17		0.001-0.920†
	0.006-0.514†		0.01-0.13
Female	0.006-0.038	Women, venous	0.06-1.44
Heart	0.002-0.078†	Menstrual	0.18
	0.001-0.016	Serum	0.000-0.0028
Liver	0.09-0.30	Skin	0.009-0.59†
Kidney	0.005-0.246†	Urine	0.01-0.22
	0.07-0.14		0.000-0.11
Pancreas	0.002-0.363†	Uterus	0.010-0.188†
	0.07	Membrane	45.6
	0.005-0.410	Aorta	0.003-0.570
Bladder	0.06	Adrenal	0.002-0.293†
Stomach	0.04	Breast	0.30-0.221†
Contents	0.003-0.104†	Muscle, pectoral	0.12-0.431†
		Ovary	0.013-0.260†
		Prostate	0.010-0.090†

*(National Research Council, 1977
†Dry weight.

samples of natural materials. The book lists 892 scientific references on arsenic (National Research Council, 1977).

Arsenic Content of Tissues from Poisoning Victims

There have been a number of documented cases of arsenic poisoning in man with the sources known and the amount of poison found in various tissues also known (National Research Council, 1977). For example, a number of industrial poisonings with arsenic have been recorded in the scientific literature. In such cases, the amount of arsenic in the hair of the victims varied from 0.4 to 816.0 of arsenic on a fresh weight basis. In similar industrial exposures, the amount of arsenic found in the urine varied from 0.04 to 0.9 ppm. In a number of cases where the source of arsenic is listed generally as "pollution," arsenic in hair has been recorded at a level of 3.6 ppm. In the thyroid gland, arsenic was found in amounts of 0.002 to 0.093 ppm.

The results of a number of exposures to arsine have been reported, and the following concentrations in various tissues are recorded in ppm of arsenic with reference to fresh weights of tissues: brain, 1.0 to 1.4; lung, 2.3 to 2.6; liver, 4.4 to 6.9; kidney, 0.4 to 1.3; stomach, 0.1 to 0.3; and spleen, 0.5 to 2.2.

A few cases are listed merely as "poison." The arsenic content of tissues reported, again in ppm of fresh weight of tissue, is as follows: esophagus, 168; lung, 20; heart, 64; liver, 12.8 to 143; left kidney, 15.8 to 92; right kidney, 81; pancreas, 94; gall bladder, 41; stomach walls, 5 to 426; stomach contents, 5 to 8.84; small intestine, 132; large intestine, 259; spleen, 13; blood, 20 to 130; and urine, 27.

A few patients have been reported suffering from arsenic polyneuritis. Arsenic concentration in their fingernails varied from 7 to 18 ppm fresh tissue. One report of arsenic poisoning as a result of aerosol treatment gave values of 0.82 to 3.0 ppm arsenic in the blood. One case in which an individual was fed arsenic showed blood values varying from 0.83 to 0.27 ppm.

It is evident that the amount of arsenic in individuals who have been exposed by some route to arsenic is significantly higher than one would anticipate from the normal ranges shown in Table 9-I. It is also worthy of comment to point out that, despite the fact that arsenic has been around for a long time as a poison, detailed information on the concentration of arsenic in the various tissues of arsenic-poisoned victims is remarkably incomplete. All tissues have not been studied; the tissues that have been studied are spread throughout the literature and associated with various routes of entry or sources of exposure in such a manner as to make generalizations difficult.

Toxicity of BAL

As is true for any chemical introduced into the human body, BAL itself, although an antidote for some metallic poisonings, is also a poison. Ordinarily, toxic signs are found when more than 4 to 5 mg of BAL per kg of body weight are given. At doses higher than this, about 15 to 20 minutes after the injection, vomiting, severe lacrimation (shedding of tears), salivation, and elevated blood pressure are usually observed. These signs of poisoning can usually be controlled by the careful administration of barbiturates. The signs and symptoms of BAL poisoning show much the nature of serum sensitivity.

Mercury

Inorganic mercury exerts poisoning action primarily by its corrosive action on tissues of the body such as the mouth and the lining of the digestive tract. Nevertheless, inorganic mercury is absorbed if swallowed and ends up in internal organs, where it can cause damage. Table 9-II may be useful.

Organic mercury is readily absorbed by the body and is severely poisonous. One case comes to mind of a worker who inhaled organic mercury fumes for five years. Signs and symptoms of poisoning developed rapidly at the end of that time, followed by death in one month. Mercury in major body organs (ppm) obtained at autopsy was: liver, 14 kidney, 3; and brain 3 to 10 depending on location.

A similar case involved a worker who breathed methyl mercury fumes for 3 years. Toxic signs and symptoms developed rapidly at the end of that time, with death resulting in two months. Organ levels of mercury in this victim (ppm) were: liver, 39; kidney, 27; and brain, 12.

Table 9-II
MERCURY POISONING

Source of Mercury	Amount (ppm)		
	Liver	*Kidney*	*Brain*
1. 50-year-old male dead 3 days after swallowing mercuric chloride	32	70	2
2. 18-year-old female dead 6 days after swallowing mercuric chloride	3	16	1
3. Mercuric chloride death, no details	68	144	1
4. 32-year-old male dead 7 days after drinking 10 gm mercuric chloride in water	30	28	0.2

In the cases of Minamata disease (methyl mercury) in Japan, the organ content varied depending on the length of exposure: liver, 26 to 38 ppm, kidney, 29 to 39 ppm; and brain, 5 to 15 ppm.

As a generalization victims of obvious organic mercury poisoning will show signs and symptoms as follows:

Virtually all victims have:

> Paresthesia, constriction of vision, hearing loss, speech disorders, muscle disorders, defective handwriting, unsteady gait

More than one-half of them have:

> Psychological disturbances, tremor, inability to stand erect with eyes closed

One-third may show:

> Excessive salivation, excessive sweating, rigidity, irregular spasmodic movements, purposeless jerky movements of arms and legs, exaggerated muscle stretch reflexes, pathological reflexes

Pathological examination confirms the view that most damage of concern from organic mercury compounds is done to the brain.*

---

*A study of cadavers (corpses) of persons from northern Colorado, ranging in age at death from one to ninety years, revealed no trend of elevated lead or mercury in body organs with the passage of time (Schmidt and Wilber, 1978). Comparison of the organ mercury levels found in the present study with values for tissues collected at autopsy sixty years ago indicates that the mercury content of most organs has decreased sharply over the past six decades.

Thallium Poisoning

Thallium is a poison used for control of unwanted wildlife such as coyotes and various wild rodents. It is also used from time to time to eradicate other forms of animal pests. Accidental poisonings do occur in man, but not so frequently as in the past when thallium was used in various hair-removing preparations (Bank et al, 1972).

The metal thallium was discovered in 1861 by Crookes using spectroscopic methods. He was examining the residues of selenium that had been obtained during the manufacture of sulfuric acid and in the process of his studies, came upon this unknown new element. In 1862, Lami isolated thallium and obtained its properties as an element (McNamara, 1944).

Patients who for some reason have received approximately 8 mg of thallium per kg of body weight completely lose all head hair after approximately two weeks. This characteristic of thallium resulted in a rather widespread use of thallium salts in Europe as a systemic depilatory in fungus diseases of the human scalp. Very shortly after the discovery of thallium, it became popular in the United States as a paste for depilatory use and also as a poison for rats. The rather careless use of thallium for those purposes resulted in a large number of accidental poisonings and fatalities.

Clinical Signs and Symptoms

There are numerous reports describing the signs and symptoms of thallium poisoning (*Clinical Toxicology,* 1972). In general, mild cases result in some pains in the joints, drowsiness, and lack of appetite. Alopecia (baldness) results after about two weeks. As a general rule, complete recovery and regrowth of the hair occurs. If the degree of poisoning with thallium is moderately severe in man, there is first pain and weakness in the lower extremities and paresthesia (abnormal sensation) and hyperesthesia (excessive sensitivity) occur in the legs and sometimes in the arms. Frequently, pain is experienced in the chest region and in the joints. The victims of such poisoning are listless and constipated and usually complain of cramps in the abdominal area that may be quite violent. The signs and symptoms run a course of several weeks; loss of hair begins during the first or second week. There are some laboratory findings that seem important: a slight leucocytosis and a mild degree of albumin and thallium in the urine.

In severe thallium poisoning, within 24 hours after the poison has been taken by a man, vomiting, paresthesia, and severe cramps occur. Salivation increases and inflammation of the mouth region becomes marked. Blebs occur on the lips; in some of these poisoning cases, a purple line may be seen at the gum line. All victims of severe thallium poisoning exhibit signs of brain damage; these signs include choreiform (jerky) movements, twitching, convulsions, and delirium; these signs of brain damage develop within five days after the poison has entered the body. Just before death in these cases, the body temperature rises significantly, from about 102.8°F to as high as 108.2°F. There is significant individual variation in the fever development. Death is apparently the result of respiratory failure.

Pharmacology

Thallium is poisonous to man in all its actions. The monovalent salts of thallium are about 10 times more poisonous than are the trivalent compounds of thallium. Thallium acetate in the amount of approximately 8 mg of the thallium salt per kg of body weight has been used as an oral depilatory. If the dose is reduced to 6 mg of thallium acetate per kg of body weight, if is not effective. On the other hand, a dose of 10 mg acetate per kg of body weight is clearly poisonous. It once was maintained that adults are more susceptible than children to thallium poisoning. There seems to be little substance for this claim. It is also known that repeated small doses of thallium produce toxicity through an accumulative action.

Cumulative Poison

According to Hayes (1963), "Thallium is a cumulative poison. The repeated dose necessary to produce toxicity is not so well known. The daily oral administration of thallium acetate to rats in less than 1/50 of the single LD_{50}-dose caused depilation in 6 weeks and death in rats within 4 months. The threshold limit for thallium in the air is 0.1 mg./M^3."

The depilatory action of thallium is a useful diagnostic sign of thallium poisoning. Thallium is no longer accepted, at least in the United States, as a component in depilatories to be used by human beings.

Effects of Thallium

THE CENTRAL NERVOUS SYSTEM EFFECTS. Thallium has a powerful destructive effect on the central nervous system and on the peripheral nerves of the body. Persons who are subjected to thallium poisoning show pain, tenderness, hyperesthesia, paresthesia, and objective sensory disturbances in the extremeties. These reactions are followed by convulsions, choreiform twitchings, disorientation, delirium, and mental deterioration.

THE AUTONOMIC NERVOUS SYSTEM. The depilatory action of thallium referred to previously seems to be associated with the sympathetic nervous system. There is some controversy about this matter, however.

THE ENDOCRINE SYSTEM. A number of the effects observed in thallium poisoning has been interpreted as the result of specific action on the endocrine system.

Fate of Thallium in the Body

Thallium enters the body through the digestive tract, the lungs, and the skin. By any one of these routes, thallium is a severe poison. Thallium taken into the body appears in the urine within 2 hours after the poison has been swallowed. As suggested earlier, thallium in small doses may be stored in the body so that a cumulative effect of the poison has been documented. The elimination of thallium is primarily through the kidneys. Thus, thallium appears in the urine as long as there is any left in the body to be eliminated. Reports have been made in the scientific literature to the effect that thallium has been found in the urine anywhere from 2 to 2½ months after a single oral dose of the toxicant has been swallowed. Most tissues of the body store thallium to some degree, with the exception of fat. Experimental studies using rats indicate that the rate of elimination of thallium is approximately 0.4 mg/kg of body weight per day. There are significant variations from one person to another and with age of the individual.

In human beings poisoned by thallium, the main route of elimination is through the kidney; a small amount of the thallium is eliminated by way of the intestine. In man, only about 3.2 percent of the thallium in the body is excreted per day.

Treatment of Poisoning by Thallium

There is no truly specific antidote for thallium poisoning. At the present time, the following procedure seems to be reasonable. First, if the thallium has been accidentally or suicidally swallowed, an emetic should be given in order to empty out the stomach of any residual thallium that has not been absorbed. The thallium that has been absorbed should be fixed by injecting magnesium iodide by vein. Thallium should then be allowed to leave the body by natural means. Fluids should be forced in order to aid in the washing out of thallium, as it were. In some cases, symptomatic treatment is necessary because of the lack of any specific antidote. The forcing of fluids cannot be overemphasized. It should include the administration of calcium salts, dextrose, orange juice, and even fluids by vein.

By way of summary, the suggestions of Hayes (1963) with respect to treatment of thallium poisoning in man are useful: "Gastric lavage should be done in acute cases. Activated charcoal and potassium iodide can be given orally to reduce thallium absorption. Sodium thiosulfate may be given intravenously to inactivate any thallium in the blood, but its usefulness has not been proved. In one study, dithizon, a chelating agent, was effective in 5 out of 6 severely ill children in an oral dosage of 10 mg/kg twice a day for 4 days or longer. The mechanism of action was unknown. It is generally felt that EDTA or BAL are not useful in the treatment of thallium intoxication. However, there are reports of improvement after the administration of BAL. In animals, BAL has not been effective, while dithizon (diphenylthiocarbazone) was protective in rats after thallium administration.

In one report, trihexyphenidyl (Artane) caused a striking reduction of tremors."

Background Information for Law Enforcement

The first criminal poisoning case involving thallium occurred in 1928. In 1964, one American toxicologist referred to thallium as a social menace in America. It should be recalled that these cases referred to were only criminal cases and, in view of the fact that crime is so grossly underreported, it seems obvious that many more cases of thallium poisoning in criminal activity probably occur. In fact, in certain parts of the world, thallium still seems to be a major device for a murderer (Irvine and Johnson, 1974).

Experienced clinical toxicologists maintain that "thallotoxicosis is a serious illness with long-term consequences. The problem with thallium is, that like many other poisons before it—for example, arsenic—it has a low fatal dose of only 1 to 2 g for an adult and has no apparent taste" (Curry, 1972).

There are numerous sensitive and highly reliable tests for thallium in blood, other body fluids, and tissues of the human organism. The fact that thallium can be revealed analytically by atomic absorption spectrometry makes the identification and quantitation of thallium in biological materials much less laborious than it was only a few years ago (Wawschinek et al., 1968).

In the normal human body, thallium concentrations are found in various tissues at the level of nanograms per gram of body tissue. Individuals who are poisoned with thallium have an intake of several grams. Moreover, the metal is excreted slowly. Thus, significant amounts of the toxic metal are held in the body. The ranges of thallium values found in persons poisoned with the metal are mg of thallium per 100 g of tissue. The interpretation of analytical data should not cause much difficulty.

The detection of thallium* in a dead body is sufficient reason

---

*"If the laboratory has access to an atomic absorption spectrophotometer and *also* has access to a thallium lamp, the answer can be obtained in seconds and hundreds of tissue analyses can be done per week, direct aspiration can reveal obvious cases immediately and dramatically" (Curry, 1972).

to suspect thallium as the cause of illness and death which may, of course, be accidental, suicidal, or homicidal.

THE ANALYSIS OF BIOTIC MATERIAL FOR HEAVY METALS IN SMALL CONCENTRATIONS†

The analysis of biological materials for heavy metals has always been a tedious process, especially if reasonably accurate quantitative results are desired. With the development of the atomic absorption spectrophotometric (AA) procedure, metal analyses became less time-consuming. Laborious preparation of materials and extraction of the metals in a form that could be subjected to analytical procedures was no longer necessary. "The introduction of atomic absorption analysis in toxicology has been undoubtedly the major factor in providing rapid, reliable, and easy to perform analyses that have, to a very great extent, made a new chapter in the history of detection of this class of poisons. The days in which the toxic metals (such as arsenic, thallium, lead, and mercury) provided the bulk of the work are largely being superseded by what were then unusual, if not impossible, cases to analyse" (Curry, 1972).

However, the method proved to be useful primarily for a small number of metals to be analyzed in a given sample. Although some sixty elements can be identified by the methods, the procedure does not lend itself to mass screenings of multiple metals.

Moreover, there has been an attempt in some quarters to handle the method as if it were a routine procedure analogous to a clinical test for blood sugar. It is this lack of understanding of technical pitfalls associated with the method that is of concern to the forensic scientist.

In this report, an attempt will be made to illustrate some of the limitations of the atomic absorption method. In the process, we are in no way attempting to downgrade this most useful analytical system, nor to call into question its value for the forensic scientist; we merely wish to call attention to the dangers of using the method in a way that it is not designed for, in expecting too

---

†This section written by Charles G. Wilber, William Word, Jerry Edde, and Terry Short.

much from the method, in treating the procedure as a simple, routine laboratory operation.

Installation

One cannot go to a scientific supply house and purchase an atomic absorption system like one can a case of beakers or a centrifuge and then expect to get to work with the new instrument immediately. There are many good instruments on the market, but competition is keen and the salesmen are vigorous. One must spend endless hours going over brochures and talking to salesmen before it is possible to specify a purchase.

It is extremely difficult to get clear and unequivocal statements about performance, parts, accessories, service, lifetime, or similar considerations from company representatives. The best way to get an evaluation of a piece of AA equipment in the context of needs is to consult with several fellow scientists who have such items. Their experience will be of great value.

Delivery dates are hard to control; we have found that if our bid makes such delivery dates firm and builds into the bid an automatic cancellation in the event of failure to deliver, the items seem to arrive on schedule.

Installation should be done by a factory representative or engineer, as they are sometimes called. Do not expect too much from such personnel. They are faithful but not always familiar with the latest advances in the field or with the latest bugs and modifications in their own equipment. A recent installation of an atomic absorption system with graphite rod furnace used three months from the time of delivery until the system could be put "on line" with any degree of confidence. Downtime for repairs and parts replacement must be considered and can amount to 10 percent of the usable time.

Some General Considerations

The analysis of biotic materials for heavy metals is sensitive in the extreme to contamination from a variety of sources. A basic consideration in heavy metal analyses is the elimination as completely as possible of all potential contamination.

In our experience, metals are ubiquitous; they are found in amounts sufficient to confuse analytical results and the subsequent interpretations unless measures are taken to control contamination. Lead is one of the metals found on virtually all surfaces, in reagents, and on instruments. Mercury, too, is found in unexpected places and can contaminate analytical results.

Another problem of some significance is the reverse of the contamination problem. Solutions of metals held for any length of time in various containers tend to have the metals "plate out" on the walls of the containers unless adequate precautions are taken to prevent the action. Glass storage containers are especially unsatisfactory in this regard. If the metal solution, whether standard or unknown sample, is kept strongly acid and stored in one of the modern plastic bottles, unacceptable losses of the metal from plating out can usually be obviated.

As a general procedure, *acid washing* of all instruments is the key to quality control of the analyses. In our procedures, all reaction vessels and storage containers are boiled in nitric acid before use. All acid used in the analyses is redistilled from glass stills. In turn, the glass distilled water is run through two deionizing columns before it is used.

Only stainless steel instruments are used in any of the necropsy procedures. A significant cost results from the rather rapid wearing out of stainless steel knives, scissors, forceps, and like instruments because of the strong acid treatments to insure that surface contamination is reduced to the minimum.

Preservation

In our experience, the only satisfactory method of preserving animal tissues for metal analyses is by freezing. We have tried using alcohol, formalin, and acetone; none is completely satisfactory for preservation. We, therefore, are of the strong opinion that tissues for metal analyses should be removed from the body, put into a plastic bag, sealed, and then frozen on dry ice. Later the specimen can be kept in a commercial deepfreeze. We have kept such tissues as brain, liver, and kidney under these conditions for twelve months without change in the metal values found upon analysis.

We have used, as plastic storage bags, the commercial Whirl-Pak® items, Ziploc® bags, and strong storage bags found in any food store. All serve equally well and seem to be equally free from metal contamination.

Digestion

There are arguments in the scientific literature about the relative merits of doing direct wet digestions of tissues for metal analyses, the production of an ash and then dissolving the ash in acid, and the lyophylization (freeze-drying) of the tissue with digestion of the resulting dried powder in acid. We have found that as a general procedure, the latter process is to be preferred. It has now become a routine matter in our laboratory to freeze-dry animal tissues, digest the dry powder in acid, and use the acid digest for analysis in the atomic absorption spectrophotometric system. Organs are placed individually into 25 ml Erlenmeyer flasks and then lyophylized using a twelve-part freeze-drying apparatus. Dry samples of about .1 to 2.5 gm are weighed into 16 ml polystyrene screw-capped test tubes. Concentrated redistilled nitric acid in the amount of 1 ml is added to each tube. In the series are included four empty tubes that are spiked with known amounts of the metal under analysis.

Digestion is then carried out in three steps. First, there is a two-hour digestion period carried on at room temperature with the tubes left loosely capped. Secondly, there is an overnight digestion period in which the tubes are tightly capped and put into a water bath held at 55°C. Finally, there is a two-hour period during which the loosely capped tubes are held at 55°C in the water bath with 5 ml of the especially distilled water added. We have found it desirable after adding the distilled water to tighten the cap on the tube, thoroughly shake the tube, then loosen the cap, and return the tube to the 55°C water bath for two hours.

The room temperature predigestion step must not be neglected. Failure to go through this step before heating may result in explosion of the tube; at the least, the sample will be lost. It is important when opening the hot tubes that rubber gloves and safety glasses be worn. In our laboratory, rubber gloves and safety shields in the form of glasses or chemical shields to cover the face are mandatory in all operations involving acid digestion.

After the third digestion period is completed, the tubes are re-moved from the water bath, and the samples as well as the stand-ards are filtered through acid-washed Whatman No. 541 hardness ashless filter paper into identical new, clean 16 ml plastic tubes. The material in these tubes is then ready for analysis using the atomic absorption system.

An important advantage in this system of preparing samples for analysis is the fact that the dried powder has virtually an in-definite shelf life at room temperature; it serves as a store of tissue for subsequent backup analyses should they be necessary. If the analytical results are challenged, one can always go back to the dried preparation for another sample and a confirming analysis.

Solid Sampling

We have experimented with the process of "solid sampling" as a variation that might have some advantages in cutting the time needed for analyses using the atomic absorption system. Essentially, this process is the introduction of a precisely weighed, small sam-ple of biotic material directly into the graphite tube of the graph-ite furnace, which replaces the flame in the atomic absorption system. The material is then incinerated directly, and the metal of concern is activated and read as usual by the system. We are impressed with the potential of this variation in methodology, but we are still not persuaded that it can be used widely on anything resembling a routine basis at this time.

Standards

The National Bureau of Standards sells bovine liver and or-chard leaves that contain specified amounts of heavy metals. These standards are well worth the cost of purchase and should be run along with the unknowns and the in-house analytical standards on a random basis to insure quality control. Reagent blanks must be part of every run.

The Bomb

An interesting development in analytical procedure for metal analysis is the stainless steel "Teflon®-lined" bomb. Material to be digested is put into the bomb with strong mineral acid, and the device is heated; thus, a combination of heat and high pressure aid in digestion of the sample. We have used the bomb technique on animal tissues of various kinds, plant tissues, and abiotic materials such as soil, ash, and coal.

In our experience, the bomb has been of no significant advantage in the digestion of plant or animal tissues. Soils usually digest adequately without the bomb technique, although soils heavy in sand and quartz are somewhat refractory to the digestion process. In some instances, soils may be more readily reduced to soluble form with the aid of the bomb.

At times, skin and hair may resist digestion. In these instances, the bomb does have some merit. We have found special use for the bomb in the analysis of coal. Coal is a nuisance to analyze; the bomb technique alleviates much of the problem. As indicated previously, however, for most animal tissues, we have not been convinced that the pressure bomb is essential in most laboratory procedures.

A word of caution is in order. The combination of strong acid and organic materials in the bomb with the subsequent elevation of temperature and pressure creates an explosive system. It is imperative that only small amounts of organic material be put into the bomb. We find that 1 gm of sample is the maximum safe amount. This assumes, with biological samples, 1 gm on the basis of wet weight or fresh weight. If dry weights are used, then we recommend as the maximum amount of biotic material only 0.1 of a gm in the bomb; for coal, 0.1 of a gm is the safe amount. Coal digests thoroughly using the bomb technique, and the digest is readily handled in the atomic absorption system.

Matrix

In our work and in similar studies made by others using the atomic absorption system, it soon became apparent that the matrix in which the analyzed metals occur has a significant effect on the values found.

Serious analytical errors can result if the matrix constitution of the unknown sample and that of the reference standard are not fairly similar. The use of a standard orchard leaf preparation as a reference standard when analyzing human liver for metals is not acceptable. This matrix phenomenon is not dependent on the amount of metal found in the sample; it seems to occur with the following metals; copper, iron, aluminum, barium, manganese, nickel, calcium, tin, chromium, zinc, lead molybdenum, and cadmium. This source of error becomes quite pronounced in the analysis of fish tissue for mercury. False high values are all too frequently recorded unless the reference standard is especially designed for use with fish tissues. There are a number of glaring examples of strange values for mercury in fish that can be explained on no other rational basis than a confusion of the data because of neglect of matrix influence. In areas of uncertainty such as this, one is well advised to use the method of standard additions in order to be certain that the results are representative of what is in the sample and not an artifact caused by disparity of matrices.

Standard Additions

In our experience, we have not found it necessary to use the dithizone colorimetric method to standardize our atomic absorption procedures. It is fortunate that the National Bureau of Standards provides a liver preparation containing specified amounts of various metals as a reference for establishing baselines. Hopefully the National Bureau of Standards will make available other reference standards for metals such as fish tissue, brain, and blood.

We have found that the method of standard additions is important if we are to examine a tissue with an unknown amount of metal in it, especially if the level of concentration of the metal is low. Essentially, the method of standard additions involves the spiking of the unknown with a precisely known quantity of metal under consideration. In such an analysis, we use three separate concentrations of the spike. A straight line is then obtained when absorbance is plotted against concentrations of the metal. When this line is carried down to 0, one can then estimate the exact amount of metal in the sample. Ordinarily, we find this method vital when working with liver. Liver provides a complex and confusing matrix. In our estimation, the method of standard additions is the method of choice to overcome the complex liver matrix.

Many laboratories use direct aqueous comparisons in which a known sample is run through the atomic absorption procedure along with the unknown. Then by direct cross comparison, it is possible to estimate the metal in the unknown using an appropriate calibration chart. Unfortunately, if the matrix in which the metal occurs is as complex as one finds in liver, the direct aqueous comparison is sometimes misleading (Table 9-III) .

Table 9-III

MINIMUM LETHAL DOSE OF COMMON METALS FOR A 160 POUND MAN
(Single acute doses)

Metal	Minimum Lethal Dose
Antimony	2 gm
Arsensic	200 mg
Beryllium	100 mg/cu. m
Bismuth	15 gm
Cadmium	1 gm
Copper sulfate	8 gm
Lead salts	10 gm
Lead tetraethyl	100 mg
Mercuric chloride	500 mg
Silver nitrate	2 gm
Thallium	500 mg
Yellow phosphorus	200 mg
Zinc sulfate	5 gm

SELENIUM AND HUMAN HEALTH*

Selenium, a metalloid, was first shown to be of practical importance in biology in the 1930s, when it was discovered that consumption of plants containing excessive quantities of this element was responsible for "alkali disease" and "blind staggers," two maladies that afflict livestock in certain areas of the Great Plains of the United States. We now know that the soils in these regions

*A statement of the Food and Nutrition Board Division of Biological Sciences Assembly of Life Sciences National Research Council (Prepared by the Committee on Nutritional Misinformation, National Academy of Sciences, September, 1976.

contain high levels of selenium in a form that is readily available for uptake by the plants eaten by grazing animals. Signs of chronic selenium poisoning generally observed in farm animals include growth depression, loss of appetite, emaciation, lack of vigor, stiffness of the joints, loss of hair, cracking of the hoofs, impairment of reproduction, anemia, and fatty liver degeneration that ultimately results in hepatic cirrhosis. Signs of selenosis noted in people living in seleniferous areas include loss of hair, brittleness of fingernails, garlic odor of the breath, and indefinite sociopsychological effects such as fatigue and irritability. Chronic selenium toxicity is seen in animals after weeks or months of ingesting plant materials that contain 5 or more ppm of selenium. On this basis, overt chronic selenium intoxication would be expected in human beings after long-term consumption of 2400 to 3000 μg daily.

In 1957, selenium was shown to have a beneficial nutritional effect in that it prevented dietary liver necrosis in vitamin E deficient rats. Very soon thereafter, selenium was shown to be of value against several vitamin E related nutritional deficiency diseases in a wide variety of species. Selenium and vitamin E had in common the fact that each offered similar protection against a perplexing array of nutritional disorders that involved the liver, skeletal and cardiac muscle, and the vascular system. More recently, selenium was established as an essential nutrient independent of vitamin E, since animals fed highly purified diets responded favorably to selenium supplements even when given adequate levels of vitamin E. The relationship between selenium and the antioxidant role of vitamin E, which puzzled investigators for many years, has now been satisfactorily explained by the discovery that glutathione peroxidase, an enzyme that detoxifies products of oxidized fats, is a selenium-containing enzyme.

The amount of selenium needed to prevent deficiency diseases in animals is very small; 0.1 ppm in the diet is a nutritionally adequate level for most species. Such a level translates into a human requirement of about 60 to 120 μg/day, depending upon the biological availability in the diet, a person's physiological status with regard to other nutrients, and other factors.

Available evidence suggests that a well-balanced American diet furnishes this quantity of selenium. Estimates of typical selenium intakes in the United States average about 150 $\mu g/day$, and diet composites analyzed in Canada provided 98 to 220 $\mu g/day$. Organ meats, muscle meats, and seafoods are our best sources of selenium in the diet. Grains and grain products also can contribute significant quantities of selenium, although the selenium content of these foods depends heavily on where the grains were grown. There is also considerable variation in the selenium content of eggs and dairy products. Fruits and vegetables are generally poor sources of selenium, but some exceptions to this rule include garlic, mushrooms, and asparagus.

The uneven distribution of selenium in the soils of the United States could conceivably cause persons living in low-selenium areas and consuming only locally produced foods to develop a low selenium state, just as some who live in high-selenium areas may ingest excess selenium. Such differences in the geochemical occurrence of selenium have caused some epidemiologists to postulate that an increased incidence of certain diseases observed in human populations residing in certain regions may be associated with low levels of selenium in the soil. These epidemiological associations have led to the promotion of selenium as a cure-all for a variety of human illnesses such as cancer, heart disease, sexual dysfunction, arthritis, various infectious diseases, heavy metal poisoning, weak eyes, skin and hair problems, and aging. But most nutritional authorities agree that there is currently no evidence of selenium deficiency in human populations in the United States, probably because of interregional food shipment that characterizes our present-day food supply. In addition, recent legislation that allows farmers to add selenium to the feeds of swine and poultry should help to maintain the amount of selenium in our food supply at an adequate level. Therefore, there is no justification at this time for the use of selenium supplements by the general population. Should selenium supplements eventually be considered desirable for those persons living in low-selenium areas or for those consuming vegetarian diets, a daily supplement of 50 to 100 μg could probably be taken safely.

Summary

Selenium is an unusual trace element, since both toxicities and deficiencies are known to occur in animals in the United States under natural conditions. Such extremes in the selenium intake of animals are due to the fact that the plants consumed by the animals are often of local origin and there are great geographical variations in the amount of selenium in the soil available for uptake by the plants.

In contrast to animals, the human population generally draws its food from several different regions of the country. There is no evidence at this time to suggest that the food supply in the United States contains either too little or too much selenium. There is reason, however, to suspect that indiscriminate selenium supplementation of the diet is potentially hazardous. A well-balanced diet is the best way to obtain not only selenium, but all of the other nutritionally essential trace elements as well.

Selenium References

Hoekstra, W.G.: Biochemical function of selenium and its relation to vitamin E. *Fed Proc, 34:*2083-2089, 1975.

Levander, O.A.: Selenium and chromium in human nutrition. *J Am Diet Assoc, 66:*338-344, 1975.

National Research Council, Agricultural Board, Committee on Animal Nutrition, Subcommittee on Selenium (J.E. Oldfield, Chairman): *Selenium in Nutrition.* Washington, D.C., National Academy of Sciences, 1971

Chapter 10

MISCELLANEOUS POISONS

Organic Phosphates

A s a result of intensive work in synthetic chemistry carried out by German scientists immediately before and during World War II, a new group of poisonous substances was made available for human utilization. The German chemists were searching for a class of chemicals that could be manufactured in Germany from raw materials available even in the face of the blockade of imports the British Navy would impose on Germany in the event of war. Such a blockade would cut off the reliable supply of natural insecticides the German Army would need to support military operations in such places as the African desert.

The German scientists focused their attention on a group of chemicals known as organic phosphates. They soon discovered that these chemicals were not only effective killers of insects, but they were also among the most poisonous of known substances to warm-blooded animals (Wilber, 1966).

After the termination of World War II, these compounds were discovered by the Allied forces. Chemists around the world continued to work on them; hundreds of variations in chemical structure were synthesized.

The organic phosphates all have a similar basic chemical structure; they all are built around phosphoric acid. Their mechanism of toxic action in animals is essentially the same for all chemicals in the group. The individual agents in the group of organic phosphates vary one from another in innate toxicity, rate of absorption into the body, and other biological effects.

Absorption

Organic phosphates enter the body readily through the skin, by way of the respiratory system, and through the gastrointestinal tract. Absorption through the skin is slower than the other routes but is still effective in the overall toxic potential of this class of chemicals. If the environmental temperature is high, absorption through the skin is enhanced. If the skin is broken or suffers from dermatitis, passage of these poisonous chemicals occurs more easily through the skin.

Mechanism of Action

These poisons are sometimes referred to as anticholinesterase agents because of their basic mechanism of toxic action. They all act to inhibit or put out of action the enzyme cholinesterase, which is essential for the functioning of the nervous system. This inhibition may be irreversible or reversible or somewhere between the two extremes depending on the specific organic phosphorus agent concerned. All tissues of the body contain cholinesterase, but the cholinesterase of the different tissues is not equally affected by the organic phosphates.

The rate at which the cholinesterase is depressed by a dose of one of these poisons seems to be important in the overall toxic results. The faster the rate of inhibition of the body's cholinesterase, the more severe will be the toxic response in general. A very slow depression of the blood cholinesterase levels can result from repeated mild exposures to an anticholinesterase agent without toxic signs/symptoms, even at extremely low levels of cholinesterase.

Human Signs and Symptoms

The symptoms of anticholinesterase poisoning in man include headache, dizziness, nervousness, blurred vision, weakness, nausea, cramps, diarrhea, and discomfort in the chest. The signs of poisoning are sweating, miosis (contraction of pupil of the eye), tearing, salivation, other profuse secretions from the respiratory tract, vomiting, cyanosis (blue coloration), papilledema (excessive fluid in the eye), uncontrollable muscle twitching, convulsions, coma, loss of reflexes, and loss of sphincter control (Hayes, 1963).

There have been at least 3 cases in which artificial respiration was required but was inadequate, so that the patient survived temporarily but showed severe brain damage as a result of the anoxia. The reason for the inadequacy of artificial respiration in different instances was delay in reaching the victim or resistance of the airway or other difficulty that could not be overcome by well-trained and well-equipped physicians. The patients gradually recovered from the specific signs of poisoning but remained comatose and tended to continue to have inadequate spontaneous respiration. Two of them showed temporary hyperthermia after the acute episode presumably as a result rather than a cause of brain injury. Death occurred 6 days to 4 weeks after onset. Extensive necrosis of the brain was present in those cases that came to autopsy (Hayes, 1963).

Laboratory Studies

In all cases of suspected poisoning by organic phosphates, whether suicidal, homicidal, or accidental, samples of blood and brain should be collected and sent to the toxicologist for analysis. The samples should not have any preservative and should be obtained before the body is embalmed or otherwise modified by morticians.

Special accurate techniques are available to measure the cholinesterase in the blood, red cells, plasma, and brain tissue (Witter, 1963). In cases of frank anticholinesterase poisoning, these tests show that the level of blood or serum cholinesterase is greatly depressed. Autopsy samples of blood and tissue show these changes, but the samples must be unfixed and unadulterated by foreign chemicals ordinarily used in embalming. Blood samples taken within a few days of death are adequate to give valid results —again assuming no embalming procedures have destroyed the value of the samples for analysis. The normal values of cholinesterase in human blood are shown in Table 10-I.

The red cell cholinesterase does not change with age. Plasma levels increase about 0.02 per decade in men; in women, about 0.04 per decade. As a general rule, a value of 0.5 or lower for cell or plasma cholinesterase is reason to suspect organic phosphorus poisoning. "For practical purposes, exposure to organic phospho-

Table 10-I
NORMAL VALUES OF CHOLINESTERASE IN HUMAN BLOOD*

	Men	Women
Red blood cells range	0.39 – 1.02	0.34 – 1.10
Mean ± S. D.	0.77 ± 0.08	0.75 ± 0.08
Plasma range	0.44 – 1.63	0.24 – 1.54
Mean ± S. D.	0.95 ± 0.19	0.82 ± 0.19

*(Hayes, 1963)

rus or carbamate insecticides is the only cause of significant depression of cholinesterase activity" (Hayes, 1963).

Autopsy Samples

The cholinesterase activity of red blood cells in the blood taken at autopsy is unchanged for a long time after death. Certainly, blood samples taken from a body up to 36 hours after death give valid results for cholinesterase activity. Samples of blood taken at autopsy and refrigerated give accurate values for cholinesterase for at least 3 weeks postmortem (Coe, 1974).

There is general agreement that if the cholinesterase activity in a postmortem blood sample is below 10 percent of the normal value, strong evidence points to death caused by an organic phosphate. Nevertheless, "the finding of activity greater than 10 percent of normal in post mortem samples does not rule out the possibility that death was caused by an organic phosphorus compound" (Witter, 1963).

Treatment

If the case of organic phosphate poisoning is severe, time is of the essence. Artificial respiration must be initiated; mechanical devices are preferred. Atropine sulfate is a specific first aid and treatment drug. After the cyanosis is cleared away by resuming respiration, 2 to 4 mg of the drug (1/30 to 1/15 grain) are injected by vein. The dose is repeated every 5 to 10 minutes until the victim shows the beginnings of atropinization (incipient atropine poisoning). The signs to watch for are dry flushed skin and heart rate elevated to as much as 140 beats per minute. Medical personnel then should give by vein 2-PAM (2-pyridine aldoxime methiodide, 2-PAM iodide, or parlidoxime iodide) : 1 gm for an adult, .25 gm for infants. After these matters have been attended to, decontamination of skin, mouth, eyes, and other parts of the body must be done as necessary.

If the poisoning is less severe, the victim is in all probability breathing spontaneously. The first move is to administer 1 to 2 mg of atropine sulfate (1/60 to 1/30 grain). The victim should be kept fully atropinized. Atropine sulfate can be given every hour up to as much as 25 to 50 mg/day. Decontamination of the body parts and removal of any contaminated clothing then follows. Medical personnel should then administer by vein 2-PAM if the victim is not responding favorably to the atropine sulfate alone.

Persons who have been poisoned with one of the anticholinesterase agents show great tolerance to atropine. Under these circumstances, up to 40 mg of atropine per day or more may be administered without inducing signs of atropine poisoning. Frequently, inadequate treatment of anticholinesterase poisoning is characterized by the administration of too little atropine, rarely because of too much atropine. "A mild degree of atropinization should be maintained in all cases for 24 hours, and in severe cases for at least 48 hours" (Hayes, 1963).

The overall chemical trauma resulting from intake of organic phosphate anticholinesterase agents is considered broadly and in detail by Wilber (1978).

Suicidal intake of parathion is relatively frequent in some parts of the world where that anticholinesterase is commonly used in agriculture or for other purposes. There is an interesting case of a disturbed male adult who took a glass of 25% solution of commercial parathion (about 100 ml). He was put in intensive care in the local hospital; atropine and toxigonin were given therapeutically. Blood samples were taken every 4 hours to follow the elimination of parathion from the body. The biological half-life of the parathion was found to be 25 hours: 25 hours after the incident of poisoning, 50 percent of the total dose of 25 gm had disappeared from the body. The victim recovered.

Chlorinated Hydrocarbons

These compounds have common chemical characteristics that put them together into a single group; first, these compounds are organic or carbon-containing, and secondly, they have chlorine in some way and at some place included in their molecular structure, In spite of these common characteristics, the individual chemicals in this group vary with respect to details of chemical structure and biological activity they have in living organisms.

A respectable body of information is known about the toxicology and pharmacology of these chemicals. However, the fundamental mechanism of biological action that these chemicals exert is not known for even one of the chemicals in this classification. Do the various individual chemicals listed as chlorinated hydrocarbons have different mechanisms of action? Are there subgroups within the chlorinated hydrocarbons that share different mechanisms of action? We do not know.

We do know that the chlorinated hydrocarbon chemicals (most of which are pesticides designed to kill unwanted forms of life) exert an action on the central nervous system. However, the specifics of this mechanism of action have not yet been revealed, either in humans or in experimental animals. There are certain general responses one observes in men and animals exposed to these chemicals. For example, large doses cause nausea and diarrhea. If experimental animals are given repeated dosages of these chemicals, microscopic changes in the liver and the kidney are observed after necropsy. In man, these microscopic changes have not been observed in ordinary poisonings with these chemicals. A single or acute large dose of chlorinated hydrocarbons taken by a man or an animal may produce lesions or damage to tissues, but these lesions are different than those found in the repeated or chronic doses.

Chlorinated hydrocarbons are soluble in the fat of the human body and the animal body. Consequently, these chemicals tend to be stored in the body fat of animals or men exposed to them. Some of the metabolic or breakdown products of these chemicals in the body are also stored in the fat. It makes no difference whether the chlorinated hydrocarbon is taken into the body in a single large dose or whether a number of successive small doses are taken in. The material is stored in the fat. As long as the materials are stored in the fat, they are physiologically inactive. This fact is concluded from animal experimentation in which it has been shown that enormous amounts of a given chlorinated hydrocarbon far beyond the fatal dose can be stored in the body fat without harm to the animal. In some cases, small amounts of these chlorinated hydrocarbons can be discovered in the milk and urine of animals or human beings exposed to them. The elimination of these compounds from the body fat is a slow process that begins only after further exposure to the chlorinated hydrocarbon in question has ceased.

The results of laboratory tests in animals and men that have been poisoned with chlorinated hydrocarbons are generally nonspecific. In most cases, the laboratory findings are negative. It is possible to show that a certain chlorinated hydrocarbon is in the stomach contents, the urine, the body fat, or even in certain other tissues. Further than that, laboratory analyses are not informative. Similarly, when the animals are subjected to pathological examination in the event of death or if human tissues and organs removed at autopsy from a victim of death by chlorinated hydrocarbon insecticides are examined, the results are essentially nonspecific.

There are some pathological responses found in men and animals killed with large doses of chlorinated hydrocarbons. These include dilation of the blood vessels and pinpoint hemorrhages secondary to convulsions, which may sometimes occur after poisoning with chlorinated hydrocarbons. In rodents, repeated doses of DDT given by mouth are followed by changes in the liver. Among these changes is an increase in size of the central lobe areas of the liver. Certain granules in the cytoplasm of the liver cells are changed; fat moves into the liver substance, and small globules of fat seen only under the electron microscope are found within the liver cells. However, according to Hayes (1963), "Similar changes occur in combination following exposure to other chlorinated hydrocarbon insecticides and occur separately following a wide variety of toxicants." These changes in the liver are restricted to rodents and are never found in human beings poisoned with these chemicals. All species studied to this time show the death of some liver cells after extremely high levels of chlorinated hydrocarbon intake. However, these necrotic changes are not specific for the chlorinated hydrocarbons.

Diagnosis

How then can one conclude that a person obviously ill and in need of some sort of treatment has been exposed to a chlorinated hydrocarbon? Hayes (1963) suggests the following: "Nervous symptoms and convulsions entirely similar to those of chlorinated hydrocarbon insecticide poisoning may be induced by a variety of economic poisons as well as by even less specific neurologic disease. If maximal symptoms are not reached within a matter of a few hours after acute exposure, then another diagnosis or some complicating factor should be sought. Even if it is known that an insecticide has been taken, the effect of the solvent should be carefully considered."

Treatment

The treatment of human beings poisoned with chlorinated hydrocarbons is essentially general. If the individual is showing convulsions, some form of sedation is necessary. Poison that may have been taken into the body by swallowing should be removed. Syrup of ipecac is a useful and effective medicine for causing vomiting and the resulting removal of any swallowed poison from the stomach. Under medical supervision, the stomach may be washed out by process of gastric lavage. Saline-type laxatives are sometimes used. Oily laxatives such as mineral oils are never used because they may facilitate the absorption of the chlorinated hydrocarbons. Any poison on the skin of the victim must be thoroughly washed away with soap and water. There are no antidotes specific for use in treating poisoning by chlorinated hydrocarbon pesticides. Once the victim is under medical supervision, phenobarbital may be given to control convulsions that originate in the central nervous system. The barbiturate is not intended to put the victim to sleep; rather, the drug is intended to return the poisoned subject to a relatively calm state. An interesting point is that the dosage appropriate for a poisoned victim may be so large as to cause anesthesia if the victim were not poisoned.

One so-called antidote that has been tried is calcium gluconate. According to some reports, it seems to control convulsions in experimental animals poisoned with chlorinated hydrocarbons. In a few cases of human poisoning, it is said to have had a helpful action. It may be used safely at the same time that sedatives are administered because the action of the calcium gluconate and the action of the sedatives are not the same. Epinephrine is never given in cases of poisoning by chlorinated hydrocarbons because under these conditions it might cause serious arrhythmias (irregularities in the beat of the heart) of such degree as to be fatal.

Table 10-II gives the single dangerous dose for man of various chlorinated hydrocarbons commonly available throughout the world.

Table 10-II
SINGLE DOSES OF CHLORINATED HYDROCARBONS

Chlorinated Hydrocarbon	Dangerous Dose
Technical lindane	30 gm
Pure lindane	7-15 gm
Chlordane	32 mg/kg
Chlordane	6-60 gm (fatal)
DDT	Not known (Very high)
Dieldrin	10-26 mg/kg
Endrin	0.2-1.0 mg/kg
Heptachlor	46 gm (dermal)
Toxaphene	46 gm (dermal)
Toxaphene	2-7 gm (oral, lethal)

In California on 23 July 1978, fifteen persons were poisoned when a load of Toxaphene in barrels was dumped on the highway and burned in an accident. Most of the poisoned victims were highway patrolmen and firemen. There were no fatalities; emergency room treatment with no overnight hospital admission was adequate for all fifteen victims (*New York Times,* 1978).

Others

DDT

"It also must be recognized that DDT is the safest compound used for vector control. Its clinical record is unbelievably good. It has caused serious illness very rarely and only following the ingestion of large amounts. According to experience in the western world, occupational injury has been confined to irritation of the skin, eyes, and throat of no greater frequency or severity than would be expected from the same exposure to inert dust. No injury to residents of sprayed houses has been confirmed. Storage of DDT and DDE is increased among spraymen, but without injury to health; storage among residents of sprayed houses is not increased above the traces caused by dietary intake in the same country" (Hayes, 1975).

Yellow Phosphorus Poisoning

Phosphorus is one of the basic elements, occurring as red or yellow phosphorus. Red phosphorus does not vaporize nor does it dissolve in water; when swallowed, it is not poisonous to man.

Yellow phosphorus, on the other hand, is a severe local and systemic poison (Simon and Pickering, 1976). It poisons cells and damages many of the body's organ systems: heart and blood vessels, liver, kidneys, and digestive tract. This form of phosphorus was once fairly common in the United States; it was found even in the heads of household matches. Now, because of legislation, it is found primarily in rodent-killing preparations.

These rodenticides contain anywhere from 2 to 5 percent yellow phosphorus. Some of the commercial products available are Patterson's Zinc Phosphide Rodent Bait,® Pearson's Rat Poison®, Stearn's Electric Brand Paste®, and Rat Doom Zinc Phosphide®.

A two-year-old male swallowed an unknown amount of rat poison containing 2.5 percent yellow phosphorus that he found in a garbage can. He vomited repeatedly and defecated black fecal masses twice; they were "smoking" and smelled of garlic. He arrived at the emergency room of a pediatric hospital 4 hours after the event. He was then unresponsive; his lips and nail beds were bluish in color (cyanotic). Vital signs were within normal range. He responded to pain. His vomited material smelled of garlic. Within an hour after arrival at the hospital, his heart and lungs stopped and he died.

A three-year-old female was brought into the emergency room about 3 hours after she swallowed a piece of bread that had been spread with an unknown amount of rat-killing paste containing 2.5 percent yellow phosphorus. Previous emergency medical care had included washing out her stomach with salt solution and mineral oil. Upon arrival, the child was unresponsive with elevated heart rate and respiratory rate. Her skin and mouth region were bluish in color. Her breath had a garlic odor. Heartbeat irregular; no spontaneous movements; responsive to pain. The usual battery of clinical laboratory tests was done. She passed a "smoking" bowel movement. About 2 hours after admission to emergency treatment she died.

In questionable cases of yellow phosphorus poisoning, one can usually conclude that poisoning took place if there is a garlic odor to the breath and vomit of the victim or to the fecal material passed. The feces tend to be black in color and to smell of garlic. Also, these appear to smoke and luminesce or shine in the dark. Yellow phosphorus is corrosive and may cause burns of the skin and around the mouth. There are no specific methods for treatment.

Therapy for yellow phosphorus poisoning includes removal of the poison from the body and supportive medical care to prevent collapse of the circulation and respiration in the early stages and, in later stages, delayed damage to vital organs such as liver and kidneys. Activated charcoal given by mouth as soon as possible after the poison is swallowed helps to absorb the poison and aid in the procedure of washing it out of the stomach.

Prevention is the most effective means of handling poisoning by yellow phosphorus.

Curare

Curare is a poison that was used in its natural form in hunting by South American natives. They coated their arrows with curare obtained from plant sources; when these arrows were shot into game animals, the animals were paralyzed and fell to the ground, where they could be recovered by the natives who used them for food.

Because of the peculiar characteristic the poison curare has for paralyzing the skeletal muscles while leaving the higher centers of the brain untouched, it was found useful as an adjuvant to various anesthetics.

It also is an effective poison that has been implicated in cases of homicide. For example, recently there is a case of a physician who was tried for reportedly killing five patients in a hospital by secretly administering to them lethal amounts of curare (*New York Times,* 1978).

This case is of particular interest because of the key role toxicologists played in the prosecution. Cross-examination of the toxicologists who had analyzed samples of drugs and tissues for curare was long, thorough, and, at times, vicious. The adversary activity in the courtroom was so vigorous that from time to time, it was necessary to order the jury out of the courtroom for extended periods of time in order that a dry run, as it were, of testimony by the toxicologists could be heard in the absence of the jury. If the judge approved, then the testimony was repeated in front of the jury.

One peculiarity arose in the course of this trial, and it dealt with the matter of a trained and experienced anesthesiologist testifying on the basis of his expert knowledge that some of the victims had indeed died of curare poisoning. The judge maintained that in one particular instance, the anesthesiologist could not arrive at the diagnosis of curare poisoning because the victim in this instance had been buried a number of years before the trial. The body had been exhumed, and only one toxicologist had reported presumptive evidence that curare was present in the body. The judge said that a second toxicologist had to confirm the findings of the first or the physician would not be allowed to testify. Some forensic scientists may look on this as a peculiar decision because the signs and symptoms of curare poisoning are unique enough to allow a skilled anesthesiologist to testify that, on the basis of his specialty, curare was the lethal agent.

Another interesting point in connection with this case is that curare was identified by the use of modern analytical techniques in bodies that had been buried for a decade. Several toxicologists using different techniques were able to identify with reasonable scientific certainty that curare actually was present in these bodies.

According to an expert anesthesiologist who testified in the case, the accused physician is said to have injected the curare into the intravenous feeding apparatus to which all five of the patients were attached. They all died suddenly. The anesthesiologist stated that in each death, there were clear indications that curare had been given by vein because intravenous curare acts most rapidly, more rapidly than by any other route.

The commercial preparation of curare, available through medical supply sources, is called *d*-tubocurarine. Ordinarily, *d*-tubocurarine is supplied as a solution in a small glass ampule. The tip of the ampule is broken off so the drug can be removed into a hypodermic syringe. The lethal effect of d-tubocurarine results from its capacity to cause paralysis of the skeletal muscles. It reacts with the particular part of the nerve cell that ordinarily responds to acetylcholine. The *d*-tubocurarine attaches to that particular location on the nerve cell so that acetylcholine cannot attach. Thus, the nerve cell cannot react. The combination of curare to the particular location is so strong that normal acetylcholine cannot break it and move in, as it were.

The action of curare is specific for skeletal muscle. It has no effect on the smooth muscles such as those in the gut or on heart muscle.

Under normal circumstances, when a skeletal muscle such as the muscles that make the ribs operate in breathing is to be activated, the nerve that supplies that particular muscle is activated by signals coming from the brain. This activation causes a nerve impulse to move down the nerve fiber toward the muscle. When the impulse gets to the end of the nerve where it approaches the muscle, acetylcholine normally is released at the nerve ending. This acetylcholine rapidly diffuses to a special location or site (called *receptor site*) on the muscle. This combination of acetylcholine and receptor causes the muscle to be activated, and it responds by contracting. When *d*-tubocurarine is present, the acetylcholine is liberated as under normal circumstances, but the *d*-tubocurarine has tied up the normal receptor sites on the muscle. Consequently, the acetylcholine cannot get there. Thus, the muscle is not activated, there is no contraction of the muscle, and such processes as movement, breathing, and so on are suppressed because the acetylcholine is crowded out from its normal tie-up with receptor sites on the skeletal muscle.

A drug such as *d*-tubocurarine is a prescription item ordinarily available only in hospitals where anesthesia of various sorts is routine. The average poisoner in our society probably would not be able to get supplies other than by breaking and entering some drugstore or medical supply house. An important point to know is that the *d*-tubocurarine in the body can be identified in the muscles, blood, liver, and kidneys. This identification is possible even after a body has been buried for a number of years.

The median lethal dose, LD_{50}, by vein for mammals varies as follows (values in mg of tubocurarine per kg of body weight) :

Dog   0.38 mg/kg
Mouse   0.11-0.15 mg/kg
Rabbit   0.165 mg/kg

The usual dose given in hospitals is 3 to 15 mg (20 to 100 units). (A unit is equal to 0.15 mg of tubocurarine.) The usual dose of the highly purified *d*-tubocurarine is 3 to 9 mg.

Neostigmine is an antidote for the toxic action of curare. It is given by vein in doses of 1 to 2 ml of a 1:200 solution, if artificial respiration with oxygen is not reviving the patient.

Acetaminophen

With the increase in the use of acetaminophen products and the apparent public opinion that it is "safe aspirin," an increase in the number of poisonings with this drug must be anticipated. For a review of the toxicity and antidotal program used, see the *Journal of International Medical Research* volume 4, Supplement 1976. This issue contains the papers presented at the "Symposium on Paracetamol and the Liver." Here are some facts. Centrilobular hepatic necrosis is dose related. Blood levels after ingestion reflect potential liver damage, that is, levels greater than 30 mg % several hours after ingestion are related to liver damage.

There are specific SH group antidotes that have been used successfully in the United States and other countries. Acetaminophen metabolites produced when toxic doses are involved bind with liver protein after glutathione is depleted. This covalent binding with hepatocytes causes the liver damage. The reason for antidotal therapy with such substances as methionine is to prevent the metabolite from binding with the liver cells *(The Toxicology Newsletter,* 1977).

The "safer than aspirin" has no anti-inflammatory action such as is desirable for arthritic persons. Aspirin has such action.

Methyl Alcohol

Methyl alcohol, methanol, or wood alcohol is a deadly poison. Methyl alcohol is sometimes used by chronic alcoholics who are for some reason or other denied access to ethanol. Children may sometimes get methanol or wood alcohol in discarded cans or in various household chemicals. The use of wood alcohol in homicides is rare but not unknown. A common source of wood alcohol is bootleg liquor, the source of which is ordinarily not known with any precision.

Methyl alcohol is insidious in its action because, as a general rule, there is a symptom-free period of 12 to 24 hours after the methyl alcohol is drunk. There is delayed onset of acidosis. Vision is disturbed. The retina and the optic nerve are damaged so that even in mild cases of methyl alcohol poisoning, the victim probably is permanently blinded if he recovers. Animal experiments are not particularly helpful in understanding poisoning with methyl alcohol.

There is no specific first aid treatment for methyl alcohol poisoning. The individual should be removed from the source of poisoning, of course. If the ingestion or swallowing of the wood alcohol has been quite recent, the victim can be induced to vomit by use of a probing finger or by administration of syrup of ipecac. Medical treatment is the only choice. According to the Armed Forces Institute of Pathology, "The old treatments of alkalinization to combat the acidosis and forced ethanol to compete for metabolic pathways are still extant. In addition, peritoneal dialysis and artificial kidney dialysis/hemodialysis have proved successful" (Kiel, 1966).

The fundamental mechanism of action of methyl alcohol poisoning is based on the chemical change of the methyl alcohol when it gets into the body to formaldehyde, which is then carried around to the various tissues of the body. Formaldehyde, of course, is a strong tissue poison. It is used in the process of embalming corpses and is also used as a preservative for anatomical specimens (Table 10-III).

Table 10-III
MINIMUM LETHAL DOSES OF VARIOUS POISONS
FOR A 160 POUND MALE

Poisons	Minimum Lethal Dose
Arsenic	200 mg
Strychnine	100 mg
Nicotine	60 mg
Aconitine	10 mg
Chloral	5 gm
DDT	>15 gm
Barbiturates	1-6 gm
Formaldehyde	50 ml
Whiskey	1 quart
Cantharidin	30 mg
Camphor	2 gm
Chlorates	8 gm
Mercuric chloride	0.5 gm
Organic phosphates	15 mg
Phenol (carbolic acid)	15 ml
Boric acid	10 gm
Cresol	8 gm
Croton oil	1 ml
"1080," sodium fluoroacetate*	50 mg

*This chemical is a severe poison that is quite hazardous because there is no known antidote for it.

Chapter 11

SOME COMMON POISONS AND
THEIR CHARACTERISTICS

L AW ENFORCEMENT officers may, during their patrol duties, encounter crises caused by the release of poisonous chemicals on
streets, roads, parking areas, railroad right-of-ways as a result of
accidents that damage tank cars or trunks, rupture cylinders of
compressed gases, or otherwise breach containers of toxic chemicals.

Phosgene

This gas is one of the outdated chemical warfare agents still
carried on the list of potential chemical agents to be used by various military groups. Industrially, it is known as carbonyl chloride
and is transported over public routes by truck or train. Carbonyl
chloride is used by the dye industry, organic chemical manufacturers, and drug companies.

It has a strong, common, musty odor. It is a severe poison,
destroying the lining of the air sacs in the lungs and allowing
body fluids to flow into the lungs. The victim literally drowns in
his own body secretions (severe pulmonary edema).

Symptoms

Symptoms consist of coughing, tightness of the chest, some
lacrimation (weeping). If exposure is severe, breathlessness, illness, and death follow.

For industrial work areas, 1 part of phosgene per million parts
of air is considered safe; 2 ppm causes nose and throat irritation.
Table 11-I may be useful.

Table 11-I
PHYSIOLOGICAL RESPONSES TO PHOSGENE

Concentration	Effect
1 ppm	Maximum allowable
1.25-2.5 ppm	Dangerous to life if prolonged exposure
5 ppm	Cough and dyspnea in 60 seconds
10 ppm	Eye, respiratory tract irritation, 60 seconds
12.5 ppm	Dangerous to life in 1-2 minutes
20 ppm	Severe lung damage in 1-2 minutes
25 ppm	Danger to life in a short time
90 ppm	Rapidly fatal

First Aid

Remove any victim from the contaminated area. Forbid even the mildest physical activity and keep the subject warm. Hospital care is mandatory as soon as possible. Oxygen should be given by mask if available. Medical treatment must be aimed at preventing the potentially fatal delayed pulmonary edema.

Liquified Natural Gas

More and more, liquified natural gas under high pressure is being transported through settled areas. Liquified natural gas can pose a hazard to human beings from two possible routes. First if spread over an area, the gas can asphyxiate individuals if the concentration is high enough. The gas itself is not poisonous; it does not contain toxic gas such as carbon monoxide. However, it does not support respiration and consequently can cause death or severe disability simply by shutting off the oxygen supply to persons enveloped in a cloud of natural gas. Secondly, and probably more importantly, is the fact that liquid natural gas burns readily. When it is released as a result of an accident, it frequently ignites and poses a severe threat to property and lives.

Diet-Drug Interactions*

While there is considerable information known about the effect of one drug on the efficacy or metabolism of another drug, current attention is being focused on the interactions between

*This section (with minor modifications) courtesy of the National Dairy Council, *Dairy Council Digest,* 6300 North River Road, Rosemont, Illinois 60018.

nutrients in the diet and drugs. This section will review the state of knowledge regarding such interrelationships from two viewpoints: a) what the effects of drugs on nutritional status are, and b) how drug response is altered by nutrients in the diet.

A drug has been defined as "any chemical compound that may be used on or administered to humans or animals as an aid in the diagnosis, treatment, or prevention of disease or other abnormal condition, for the relief of pain or suffering, or to control or improve any physiologic or pathologic condition." A nutrient, on the other hand, refers to a substance that affects the nutritive or metabolic processes of the body. Present in the daily diet or used to supplement an inadequate diet, a nutrient functions to prevent a disease caused by an inadequate intake of the particular nutrient. The broad definition of drugs above may encompass certain nutrients, particularly when these nutrients are used in the treatment of a disease whether causally related to inadequate dietary intake or not. For example, vitamin C has been used to acidify the urine in the treatment of bladder infections, while nicotinic acid has been prescribed to lower serum cholesterol levels. The nutritional, rather than the pharmacological, role of nutrients will be considered in this discussion of nutrient interaction with drugs.

Drugs and Nutritional Status

Factors commonly considered in the assessment of individual nutritional needs include age, body size, activity, previous and current nutrient intake, and disease conditions that affect nutrient metabolism. Gaining increasing recognition is the effect of drug therapy, particularly long-term usage and multiple drug regimens, on nutritional needs which ultimately determines nutritional status.

Numerous drugs can potentially effect nutritional status through various means. Some may alter food intake indirectly by producing side effects such as nausea, vomiting, and altered sense of taste. Some others may inhibit nutrient synthesis, and still others may interact with nutrients to reduce absorption, to alter their distribution, transport, utilization, or storage, and to increase excretion of nutrients.

How these interactions affect one's nutritional homeostasis is dependent largely on the body's reserve stores of the nutrient(s) affected, on compensatory adaptive mechanisms in nutrient absorption and excretion, and on the relative adequacy of the dietary intake of the nutrient(s). It is when the body is unable to adapt to the challenges imposed by drug therapy that gradual nutrient depletion becomes a likely outcome.

It is important to realize that by possibly accentuating pre-existing subclinical malnutrition of dietary or disease origin, drug-nutrient effects may give rise to clinical syndromes of nutrient depletion. It is equally significant to recognize the other side of the coin; that is, in some cases, maintenance of desirable nutritional status can permit use of higher dosages of therapeutically valuable drugs since the individual's tolerance for the drug is increased.

The various means by which drugs may affect one's nutritional status will be given brief consideration.

APPETITE AND TASTE. The most widely recognized example of drug-nutrient relationship is that of pharmacological agents prescribed for treatment of obesity. Most of these drugs are amphetamines that depress appetite. However, amphetamines presently offered for obesity control have not been uniformly effective nor without potential hazard; thus, the problem of obesity still lacks a satisfactory pharmacological answer.

The emotional, psychological, cultural, social, economic, and organoleptic factors that exert important effects on appetite and food intake complicate interpretation of experimental results and may account for the paucity of precise scientific data on the effect of drugs on appetite in man. However, there are drugs known to alter taste acuity or have an unpleasant taste that causes nausea and gastrointestinal upset, which in turn depress appetite. There also are those bulk agents like methylcellulose and guar gum, which take up fluid and swell in the gastrointestinal tract. Because of the resulting feeling of fullness, they may slightly reduce appetite.

On the other hand, there are drugs that may increase appetite and, thus, food intake. These include insulin, steroids, sulphonylureas, psychotropic drugs, and certain antihistamines. However, as in the case of appetite control, there is no available safe and effective drug at the present time to reliably increase appetite to a significant degree in man.

NUTRIENT SYNTHESIS. Drugs can influence synthesis of vitamins as a result of pharmacodynamic action in the cell. For example, physical as well as chemical ultraviolet light barriers may decrease vitamin D synthesis in the skin. Drugs, particularly antibiotics, can inhibit bacterial synthesis of vitamins in the gastrointestinal tract; for example, tetracyclines and other broad spectrum antibiotics can inhibit vitamin K synthesis. Chloramphenicol also has been found to decrease protein synthesis.

NUTRIENT ABSORPTION. In order to better understand the mechanisms underlying the effects of drugs on intestinal absorption of nutrients, it is important to recognize that factors involved in drug absorption differ from those governing nutrient absorption.

Absorption of drugs is dependent on lipid solubility, on rate of dissociation (pKa) and pH of medium, on particle size, and on the physical form. Generally, drugs cross the gastric and/or intestinal mucosa by passive nonionic diffusion. Drugs that are weak acids are absorbed in the stomach, those that are weak bases in the upper intestine, while neutral compounds do not have definite preference for site of absorption. Digestive enzymes are not involved, and competitive inhibition (decreased absorption of a substance caused by preferential absorption of another, using common metabolic pathways) does not appear to occur.

In contrast, absorption of nutrients depends, in large part, on the presence of gastrointestinal secretions, on pH, and on the enzymatic activity of absorptive cells. With the exception of vitamin B_{12}, the majority of nutrients is absorbed in the upper intestines through mechanisms including passive diffusion and active transport. The degree of lipid solubility is important only for fats; water-soluble nutrients are absorbed and transported by the nonlipid phase of intestinal content. Some nutrients like simple sugars and amino acids display competitive inhibition.

Groups of drugs that may cause malabsorption include the following: a) those that affect intestinal motility such as laxatives or cathartics; b) hypocholesterolemic drugs such as cholestyramine; c) biguanides used in diabetes; d) antibiotic drugs like neomycin; f) anticonvulsant drugs such as diphenylhydantoin; and g) colchicine used in gout.

Roe attributed drug-induced impairment of nutrient absorption to any one of several possible mechanisms. First, a drug can solubilize a nutrient, as in the case of mineral oil dissolving dietary carotene, which then is lost to the normal absorptive process and passes out in the feces. Second, drugs can absorb or interfere with the physiological activity of bile salts so that fats and fat-soluble vitamins that require bile salts for optimal absorption are taken up inefficiently from the intestinal tract. Third, drugs can induce cellular damage to the intestinal mucosa or selective block of and interference with nutrient transport mechanisms. Fourth, drugs can damage the exocrine pancreas, which causes decreased synthesis and/or release of pancreatic enzymes with consequent maldigestion of fat, protein, and starch.

NUTRIENT DISTRIBUTION AND EXCRETION. Drugs can either a) displace nutrients from plasma protein– or tissue-binding sites by complexing the nutrient and thus detaching it from the binding sites, b) replace the nutrient on a protein-binding site, or c) produce a combination of these effects. These interactions promote renal excretion of the affected nutrients, which can either be free or complexed with the drug.

NUTRIENT METABOLISM. The effect of drugs on the metabolism of nutrients has been the subject of numerous reviews. Eisenstein presented a detailed discussion of the effects of adrenal cortical hormones on various aspects of carbohydrate, protein, and fat metabolism. Truswell discussed the effects of drugs on lipid metabolism in terms of those that a) cause malabsorption, b) increase fecal excretion of bile acids, c) inhibit cholesterol absorption, d) affect lipoprotein lipase, e) cause fatty liver, f) affect free fatty acid release from adipose tissue, g) lower plasma lipid concentration, and h) increase plasma lipid concentration.

Marks classified drugs that affect carbohydrate metabolism into those that tend to raise and those that tend to lower the fasting blood glucose, adding that, in certain instances, the amount and circumstance under which the drug is administered determine whether it produces a rise, a fall, or no change in blood glucose concentration. Considered in his review are the mode of action and effect of drugs on glucose metabolism in man. However, he did not discuss the effects of drugs upon intermediary metabolism nor did he discuss other carbohydrates of nutritional importance such as fructose, galactose, and the disaccharides.

A number of investigations and reports have been concerned with the effect of drugs on vitamin metabolism. Drugs may function as antivitamins either by blocking the conversion of a vitamin to its coenzyme form, by inhibiting the synthesis of its active metabolite, or by promoting the retention of the inactive form of the vitamin. Structurally unrelated drugs that stimulate the activity of drug-metabolizing enzymes can also stimulate cellular catabolism and reduce body stores of fat-soluble and water-soluble vitamins. Biochemical signs and symptoms of vitamin D deficiency have been evident among children and adults on chronic anticonvulsant drug therapy.

There is clinical and experimental evidence suggesting that anticonvulsants enhance the breakdown of vitamin D by inducing hepatic microsomal enzymes. Also, because the drugs increase the conversion of vitamin D to polar inactive metabolites, it has been suggested that anticonvulsant drug induced osteomalacia may be due to the decreased levels of the biologically active metabolites of vitamin D.

ORAL CONTRACEPTIVES. The use of oral contraceptives has been associated with a number of metabolic changes suggestive of altered nutritional status with regard to several minerals such as phosphorus, magnesium, and calcium as well as vitamins including vitamin A, thiamin, riboflavin, ascorbic acid, folic acid, pyridoxine, vitamin B_{12}, and vitamin E. Although these metabolic changes suggest an association with increased metabolic needs for several nutrients, relatively few clinical correlations have been identified. Thus, until further research data become available, the Committee on Nutrition of the Mother and Preschool Child of the Food and Nutrition Board, NAS/NRC will not provide a

246 Forensic Toxicology for the Law Enforcement Officer

definitive recommendation regarding the use of nutritional supplements to oral contraceptive users.

ANTACIDS. The effect of antacids on mineral metabolism also has been reported by Spencer et al. Their studies indicated that small amounts of antacids containing aluminum inhibited the intestinal absorption of phosphorus and fluoride, caused a reversal of the urinary and fecal phosphorus excretion, and increased the excretion of calcium in urine and stool. They added that if the calcium losses caused by antacid therapy continued for prolonged periods of time, significant skeletal demineralization might occur.

Nutrient Effect on Drug Response

Variability in drug response is a major therapeutic problem; thus, it is important to determine whether normal dietary constituents stimulate or inhibit the metabolism of drugs, thereby altering their biological effects.

It cannot be generalized, however, that the mere presence of food in the alimentary tract can delay or accelerate absorption of an orally administered drug. A recent study revealed that the absorption or bioavailability of an oral dose of procainamide (used to control ventricular arrhythmias) does not appear to be significantly altered by simultaneous ingestion of food. However, it is generally recognized that food in the gastrointestinal tract causes changes in pH, motility, and gastrointestinal secretions, which in turn may affect ionization, stability, solubility, transit time, and absorption of drugs. In addition, several factors can influence the bioavailability of a drug. These include inactivation of the drug before gastrointestinal absorption, incomplete absorption, biotransformation of the drug, and the individual's physiological status.

The interactions between nutrient and drug more often than not involve the effects of nutritional imbalance on the drug-metabolizing enzymes, which will be briefly described. Drugs are removed from or detoxified in the body by a group of nonspecific enzymes that are located predominantly, although not exclusively, in liver microsomes. This hepatic microsomal drug-metabolizing enzyme system, conventionally classified as a mixed function oxidase (MFO), is comprised of the heme protein cytochrome P-450, phosphatidylcholine, and a flavoprotein reductase and requires oxygen and nicotinamide adenine dinucleotide phosphate. Because a variety of drugs appears to be metabolized, this system must possess a broad substrate "specificity."

Nutritional imbalance exerts impact on drug response by the alteration (stimulation or inhibition) of the activities of this enzyme system. The processes of metabolism and activities of this enzyme system are affected by acute starvation, undernutrition, protein nutrition, and deficiencies or excesses of minerals, vitamins, and lipids. The activity of the drug-metabolizing enzymes has been reported to decrease with diets deficient in calcium, zinc, magnesium, and ascorbic acid, while it has increased with diets supplemented with alpha-tocopherol. Lipids are essential for the proper functioning of this enzyme system because the enzymes are associated with the lipiprotein membranes of hepatic-endoplasmic reticulum, 30 to 40 percent of the dry weight of which is lipid. The effects of dietary lipids on MFO activity have been reported to depend in large part on the type of dietary fat. A dietary reduction in either quantity or quality of protein has been shown to depress MFO activities, reflecting an increased toxicity of drugs during protein deficiency.

Although the effects of nutrient imbalances on drug toxicity have been reported, one must be aware of the difficulties in assessing independently by experimentation the influence of individual nutrients. Caloric intakes and densities of the diet, stress effects, and "sparing" action that results from the supplementation of one nutrient upon the deficiency of another often are not discernible. Thus, one must be aware of the equal importance of any secondary interactions before attributing any effect exclusively to drugs.

In addition to the effect of nutrient imbalance on the drug-metabolizing enzyme and the effect of food in general on drug absorption, drug effects may be altered by the presence as trace residues of pharmacologically active substances in food. These foreign compounds can either stimulate or inhibit the hepatic drug-metabolizing enzymes. However, there are relatively fewer confirmed examples of this effect in humans in contrast to the numerous cases reported in animals. An example of such an effect was recently reported by Pantuck et al, who observed that charcoal-broiled beef, because of its polycyclic hydrocarbon content, enhanced the metabolism and lowered the plasma levels in humans of orally administered phenacetin, an analgesic antipyretic drug.

Another commonly cited interaction is that of the combination of tyramine-containing foods and monoamine oxidase inhibitors (MAOI), which results in a sudden rise in blood pressure or the so-called hypertensive crisis. Tyramine-containing foods include aged cheddar cheese, pickled herring, chianti wine, bananas, tinned and packet soups, nuts, etc. Other factors influencing the risk of such a reaction include the interval between the taking of the drug and ingesting of the food, as well as the patient's susceptibility, which may be related to his ability to metabolize tyramine. Steward stated that such factors as well as the wide variation in tyramine content of foods must be taken into account in the management of patients receiving MAOI.

There are also reports of possible decreases in drug effectiveness with the simultaneous ingestion of certain foods. For example, since tetracyclines can form insoluble complexes with calcium, magnesium, iron, and aluminum salts, the presence of food containing these salts may result in decreased or impaired intestinal absorption of these drugs. At this point, it may be prudent to emphasize the importance of strictly following label directions regarding the time when drugs may be taken in relation to mealtimes, as well as what foods may be contraindicated to take at the same time as the drugs. This raises a question as to the practice of mixing drugs with certain liquid and solid foods in an attempt to mask disagreeable taste. The pharmacological, as well as clinical, implications of this practice need to be explored further.

Cognizant of the constraints accompanying the use of human subjects for research purposes, Roe pointed to the need for prospective human studies to provide information on the incidence, etiology, and risk of drug-induced malnutrition. A comprehensive drug surveillance study among hospital patients may provide statistical relationships between biochemical indices of nutritional status and drug intake. Also needed are studies to investigate the nutritional status of populations who are on long-term medications, such as the geriatric population or women taking oral contraceptive agents.

Public health measures, for example, nutrient supplementation of common foods to reduce risk of vitamin deficiencies among oral contraceptive users, in order to control, minimize, or prevent drug-induced malnutrition remain controversial and have not to date gained widespread acceptance from the medical and scientific communities. It is imperative that those in the medical community not only be made more aware of the risks of drug-nutrient interactions but also be encouraged to support measures that will reduce the risks of drug-induced malnutrition. Among these measures are: a) avoidance of unnecessary prescriptions, b) limitations of multiple drug regimens, c) support for control of over-the-counter drug sales,* and d) dissemination of information on the nutritional effects of drugs to medical and allied health personnel as well as to the patients themselves.

Summary

Although the importance of nutritional-pharmacological interactions is not fully recognized, a better understanding of the fundamental mechanisms of these potential interactions may have valuable clinical implications in treatment of disease and malnutrition. There are a number of drugs that may affect nutrient utilization and, conversely, there are nutrients that may affect drug absorption and bioavailability. Significant differences in the activities of drug-metabolizing enzymes, which ultimately affect drug toxicity, have been shown with both adequate and deficient diets. More research is warranted to determine the mechanisms involved in nutrient-drug interactions so that risks of drug-induced malnutrition may be minimized.

---

*In a presumably democratic society, the "control" of these substances should be in keeping with individual freedoms—even the freedom of the individual to be foolish and at times uncaring about his personal health. Controls should be in the form of effective education, not arbitrary "thou shalt nots" enforced by the iron fist of penal laws. The latter approach is not appropriate in a supposedly free society and never works anyway.　　　　C.G.W.

Alcohol and Race

During its first year of operation, the Alcohol Epidemiologic Data System (AEDS) of the National Institute on Alcohol Abuse and Alcoholism has come up with findings on cirrhosis mortality rates among American Indians and blacks that may have important implications for prevention and treatment in these two minorities.

In a paper delivered at the 32nd International Congress of Alcoholism and Drug Dependence in Warsaw, Poland, it was reported:

New data indicate that the cirrhosis death rate among Indian women is almost as high as among Indian men. This is strongly suggestive of a high level of problem drinking by Indian women and points to a need for more research into the drinking patterns of this population. Previous studies of Indian alcoholism have seldom mentioned women.

Analyses of 1975 data on cirrhosis mortality rates among blacks in seven major metropolitan areas confirm earlier reports that cirrhosis death rates among blacks exceed the rates among whites. In each of the urban areas, blacks apparently tend to die from cirrhosis at a younger age and "at much greater rates" than whites.

Data pertinent to Indian women follow:
In 1975, one of four deaths among Indian women aged 35-44 was attributed to liver cirrhosis. Indian females have much higher cirrhosis mortality rates at all ages than black or white females. For example, the cirrhosis death rate for females aged 35-54 is about 125 per 100,000 persons for Indians, compared to about 39 for blacks and 15 for whites. Indian females aged 15-34 are reported to be dying of cirrhosis at 37 times the rate of white females in the same age group.

Among data pertinent to urban blacks:
The overall cirrhosis mortality rate is 44 percent higher for blacks than for whites in the seven cities studied. The cirrhosis mortality rate is significantly greater among younger members of the black populations, rising to over 10 times that of equivalent rates for whites aged 25-34. The overall ratio of black-to-white cirrhosis deaths from all seven cities in the 25-34 age groups is higher for females than for males. The ratios tend to even out for females and males at older age groups.

Orientals' Hypersensitivity

Several studies have shown that Oriental persons have a hypersensitivity to alcohol manifested after drinking by such signs as severe flushing of the skin, variable blood pressure changes, and a pounding sensation in the head.

As an explanation of this phenomenon, researchers at the University of North Carolina Center for Alcohol Studies suggest that it arises, at least in part, from acetaldehyde toxicity. A sudden buildup of acetaldehyde in the blood because of a faster initial rate of alcohol metabolism occurs when an Oriental person takes a drink, probably due to the presence of an atypical form of the liver enzyme alcohol dehydrogenase. Acetaldehyde, a by product of alcohol metabolism, has been previously shown to increase ventilation and heart rate and to cause flushing of the face after intravenous infusion, they note. Several researchers have confirmed the existence of an "Oriental form" of alcohol dehydrogenase in the liver in a majority of East Asians.

They based their conclusions on studies in 13 Occidental and 8 Oriental persons. Ethanol was given intravenously to the subjects at an "intoxicating dose" of 0.5 gm/kg during a 30-minute period and a maintenance dose of 0.15 gm/kg/hour for the next 60 minutes.

The Occidentals' mean pulse rate remained stable throughout the experiment, while the Orientals' showed an increase of about 10 percent by 30 minutes after the start of the experiment. Flushing was observed in 4 of 7 Orientals for whom data were available, but in none of the Occidentals.

Approximately $1\frac{1}{2}$ hours after the start of ethanol administration, dizziness was reported by 6 of the 13 Occidentals and in all 8 Orientals; pounding in the head was reported by 2 Occidentals and 5 Orientals; and nausea by 1 Occidental and 5 Orientals.

Breath alcohol levels were higher in the Occidentals at 15 minutes after the start of the experiment but comparable in both groups at 45 minutes. This finding was consistent with the concept that the initial rate of alcohol metabolism is faster in Orientals. Breath acetaldehyde levels were significantly higher in Oriental subjects than Occidental subjects both during and after ethanol administration.

For some time, it has been observed that the rate of alcoholism is "significantly lower" in most Orientals than in Occidentals. While this lower incidence may result partly from "cultural and psychological characteristics," it seems logical that persons experiencing dysphoria and little or no euphoria after drinking alcohol would be less prone to use the substance to excess, they said.

One puzzling observation cited is that American Indians seem to have a high predisposition to excessive alcohol use despite the same tendency as Orientals to develop high blood acetaldehyde levels after drinking. The distinctive social and cultural characteristics of Indians may account for the different reaction (National Clearing House for Alcohol Information, 1978).

What Does A Toxicology Report Mean?*

The arrival of a toxicology report often prompts a barrage of questions concerning the interpretation. Among the asked questions are the following:

1. When the toxicology request and specimens were submitted, what analyses were conducted?
2. What drugs or chemicals could or could not have been detected utilizing these analyses?
3. How accurate is the laboratory conducting these analysis?
4. Given a report that indicates the presence of a therapeutic or toxic agent, at what levels are these agents toxic and how might I find out whether or not the presence of these agents is important in causing an accident or resulting in death?

Incorporated into this section are two tables. Table 11-II presents the detection limits, methods, and degree of precision of analysis of therapeutic and toxic agents searched for in the New Mexico OMI Laboratory and lists those agents searched routinely. Included on this list are the methods whereby the drug or chem-

---

*Courtesy of James T. Weston, M.D., Editor, *Newsletter,* Office of the Medical Investigator, State of New Mexico, Albuquerque, New Mexico.

Table 11-II

DETECTION LIMITS, METHODS, AND DEGREE OF PRECISION OF ANALYSIS OF
THERAPEUTIC AND TOXIC AGENTS SEARCHED FOR IN THE
NEW MEXICO OMI LABORATORY

Drug	Qualitative Method	Quantitative Method	Detection Limits	Precision at Toxic Levels
Alcohol				
Ethanol	GLC	GLC	.002%	±8%
Methanol	GLC	GLC	.005%	±8%
Acetone	GLC	GLC	.001%	±8%
Isopropanol	GLC	GLC	.005%	±8%
Formaldehyde	GLC	GLC	.025%	±8%
Carbon Monoxide	UV	Cooximeter	2% Sat.	±5%
Phenothiazines				
Thorazine®	TLC, UV	GLC	0.2 mg/liter	±15%
Prolixin®	TLC, UV	GLC	0.2 mg/liter	±15%
Serentil®	TLC, UV	GLC	0.2 mg/liter	±15%
Trilafon®	TLC, UV	GLC	0.2 mg/liter	±15%
Compazine®	TLC, UV	GLC	0.2 mg/liter	±15%
Mellaril®	TLC, UV	GLC	0.2 mg/liter	±15%
Stelazine®	TLC, UV	GLC	0.2 mg/liter	±15%
Temaril®	TLC, UV	GLC	0.2 mg/liter	±15%
Barbiturates				
Amobarbital	GLC, UV	GLC	0.5 mg/liter	±10%
Butabarbital	GLC, UV	GLC	0.5 mg/liter	±10%
Butalbital	GLC, UV	GLC	0.5 mg/liter	±10%
Mephobarbital	GLC, UV	GLC	0.5 mg/liter	±10%
Pentobarbital	BLC, UV	GLC	0.5 mg/liter	±10%
Phenobarbital	GLC, UV	GLC	0.5 mg/liter	±10%
Secobarbital	GLC, UV	GLC	0.5 mg/liter	±10%
Stimulants				
Elavil®	TLC	GLC	.1 mg/liter	±15%
Amphetamine	TLC	GLC	.1 mg/liter	±15%
Atropine	GLC	GLC	.1 mg/liter	±15%
Desipramine	GLC	GLC	.2 mg/liter	±15%
Imipramine	GLC	GLC	.2 mg/liter	±15%
Methylphenidate	GLC	GLC	.2 mg/liter	±15%
Nortriptyline	GLC	GLC	.2 mg/liter	±15%
Pentazocine	TLC	GLC	.2 mg/liter	±15%
Strychnine	TLC	GLC	.2 mg/liter	±15%
Methamphetamine	TLC	GLC	.1 mg/liter	±15%
Tranquilizers				
Chlordiazepoxide	UV, TLC	GLC	.2 mg/liter	±15%
Diazepam	UV, TLC	GLC	.2 mg/liter	±15%

Table 11-II—(*Continued*)

Drug	Qualitative Method	Quantitative Method	Detection Limits	Precision at Toxic Levels
Ethchlorvynol	GLC	GLC	1.0 mg/liter	±15%
Flurazepam	GLC	GLC	.2 mg/liter	±15%
Glutethimide	GLC	GLC	.5 mg/liter	±15%
Meprobamate	GLC	GLC	1.0 mg/liter	±15%
Methagualone	GLC	GLC	.2 mg/liter	±15%
Methyprylon	GLC	GLC	.2 mg/liter	±15%
Oxazepam	GLC	GLC	.2 mg/liter	±15%
Narcotics				
Morphine	TLC	GLC, FLUOR	0.2 mg/liter	±15%
Codeine	TLC	GLC	0.2 mg/liter	±15%
Methadone	TLC	GLC	0.5 mg/liter	±15%
Propoxyphene	TLC	GLC	0.1 mg/liter	±15%
Meperidine	TLC	GLC	0.5 mg/liter	±15%
Pentazocine	TLC	GLC	0.2 mg/liter	±15%
Cocaine	TLC	GLC	1.0 mg/liter	±15%
Hydrocodone	TLC	GLC	0.5 mg/liter	±15%
Hydromorphone	TLC	GLC	0.5 mg/liter	±15%

ical is detected qualitatively, the methods whereby it is quantitated, the limits of detection, and the precision with which the agent is detected within the range of toxic levels. If the qualitative drug screen indicates the presence of a drug, the analysis usually proceeds toward the identification, if at all possible.

When a report indicating a negative toxicology is received back from the laboratory, it indicates the absence of those agents designated within the specific areas. Infrequently one wonders whether a drug screen conducted in another laboratory would give similar results, as though each drug screen was performed in a similar manner, using similar reagents and instrumentation. This is not the case. There are now a number of commercially available computer-linked instruments operational within many clinical laboratories which have the capability of running "drug screens" such that they might detect, within the therapeutic or toxic level, agents commonly employed as medication. In many instances, the results of such an analysis might be similar to or identical with similar analyses conducted within our laboratory, while in other instances, such an analysis might be limited to a search for only a portion of the drugs routinely searched for in our laboratory. Samples submitted for toxicology in certain cases are retained for long periods of time after their collection in the event that a representative of the defense or another litigant desires analysis by a second laboratory. For example, samples collected on homicide victims may be retained for periods of two years, while samples retained from other instances in which civil or criminal litigation is or might be contemplated may be held for at least one year after the date of death.

Table 11-III records the therapeutic and toxic levels of agents searched for in the New Mexico OMI Laboratory. This table presents the nontoxic levels that might be encountered as a result of administration of the agent for therapeutic purposes and the levels above which toxicity might be expected. Comparison of the toxic levels on this table with the possible levels of detection in the fourth column of Table 11-II indicates the difference between the limits of detection and the toxic levels. The greater the difference between the two, the greater the probability that a

Table 11-III

THERAPEUTIC AND TOXIC LEVELS OF AGENTS SEARCHED FOR IN THE NEW MEXICO OMI LABORATORY*

	Nontoxic	Toxic		Nontoxic	Toxic
Alcohol			*Barbiturates*		
Acetone	<0.01	>0.02%	Amobarbital	1-10	>20
Ethanol	0.00-0.003%	>0.400%	(Amytal®)		
Isopropanol	0	>0.08%	Aprobarbital	1-10	>20
Methanol	0	0.06-0.15%	Barbital	10-40	>60
Ether	0.05-0.13%	>0.15%	Butalbital	0.5-1.0	>10
Chloroform	0.02%	>0.02%	(Fiornal®)		
			Butabarbital	1-10	>20
Carbon			(Butisol®)		
Monoxide	<5% sat.	20-80%	Hexabarbital	0.5-1.0	>
			(Sombucaps®)		
Proprietary			Mephobarbital	10-20	>30
Acetaminophen	<10	>40	(Mebaral®)		
(Tylenol®)			Pentobarbital	0.5-1.0	>10
Acetylsalicylic	50-250	>500	(Nembutal®)		
acid (Aspirin)			Phenobarbital	10-30	>70
Chlorphenira-			(Luminal®)		
mine	.01-.02	20-30	Secobarbital	1-2	7-10
Salicylamide	10-30		(Seconal®)		
Phenacetin	1-5	>100			

Table 11-III — (Cont'd.)

	Nontoxic	Toxic		Nontoxic	Toxic
Stimulants			*Tranquilizers* (Cont'd.)		
Amitriptyline (Elavil®)	.05-.1	>1	Hydroxyzine (Atarax®)	.5	>10
Amphetamine (Benzedrine®)	.04-.3	>.5	Meprobamate (Miltown®)	5-40	50-300
Caffeine	.8-15	>50	Methaqualone (Quaalude®)	5	20
Desipramine (Norpramin®)	.01-1	>1	Methyprylon (Nodular®)	10	30-100
Imipramine (Tofranil®)	.01-.1	>1	Oxazepam (Serax®)	0.2-1.0	>2
Methamphetamine (Methdrine®)	.03-.1	>.5	Paraldehyde	30-150	500-1000
Methylphenidate (Ritalin®)	<0.1	>1	Perhenazine (Trilafon®)	0.1	>1
Nortriptyline (Aventyl®)	.01-.1	>1	Prochlorperazine (Compazine®)	0.5-2.0	5.10
Strychnine		>2	Thioridazine (Mellaril®)	0.05-0.5	>1.0
			Trifluorperazine (Stelazine®)	0.5	>1
Tranquilizers			Trimethobenzamide (Tigan®)	1-2	7-10
Chloral hydrate	<15	>100			
Chlordiazepoxide (Librium®)	1-10	15-40	*Narcotics*		
Chlorpromazine (Thorazine®)	0.05-0.5	>1	Cocaine		.1-5
Diazepam (Valium®)	.05-1	>2	Codeine	.05-.1	>1
Doxepin (Sinequan®)	<0.5	>0.5	Meperidine (Demerol®)	0.1-1.0	>5
Ethchlorvynol (Placidyl®)	5-20	>50	Methadone	.5-1	1-3
Fluphenazine (Prolixin®)	<0.5	>1	Morphine	.02-.1	>.1
Flurazepam (Dalmane®)	.05-.1	>1	Pentazocine (Talwin®)	0.1-0.5	>3
Glutethimide (Doriden®)	.5-5.0	>10	Propoxyphene (Darvon®)	0.3	>2

*All concentrations are given in mg/liter (except volatiles). It should be emphasized that these are the *usual* therapeutic and toxic concentrations, and in certain situations, the interpretation of a drug level may vary with individual circumstances.

drug or chemical in toxic levels will be detected in the laboratory. The last column in Table 11-II indicates the degree of precision in terms of reproducibility of laboratory results.

Interpretation of toxicology reports should take into consideration the degree of laboratory error that might be encountered. These may be particularly important when levels are on the borderline between the nontoxic and toxic range. Interpretation of toxicology levels in this area should be reserved for the toxicologist, as should interpretation of toxicology levels in those instances where more than one agent is reported. In many instances, the effects of the drugs are additive; in other instances, one drug tends to counteract the effect of another; while in still other instances, one drug may serve to enhance the effects of another or be synergistic. The toxicologist reporting levels considered to be significantly toxic should routinely note this interpretation on the report of the toxicologist.

Appendix I

ALCOHOL-RELATED DISORDERS*

Gastrointestinal
Esophagitis
Esophageal carcinoma
Gastritis
Malabsorption
Chronic diarrhea
Pancreatitis
Fatty liver
Alcoholic hepatitis
Cirrhosis (may lead to cancer of liver)

Cardiac
Acoholic cardiomyopathy
Beriberi

Skin
Rosacea
Telangiectasia
Rhinophyma
Cutaneous ulcers

Neurologic and Psychiatric
Peripheral neuropathy
Convulsive disorders
Alcoholic hallucinosis
Delirium tremens
Wernicke's syndrome

*(National Institute of Mental Health, 1972)

Korsakoff's psychosis
Marchiafava's syndrome

Muscle

Alcoholic myopathy

Hematologic

Megaloblastic anemia

Vitamin Deficiency Disease

Beriberi
Pellagra
Scurvy

Metabolic

Alcoholic hypoglycemia
Alcoholic hyperlipemia

APPARENT CONSUMPTION, BY STATES, OF EACH MAJOR BEVERAGE CLASS, AND OF ABSOLUTE ALCOHOL FROM EACH CLASS, IN U.S. GALLONS PER PERSON IN THE DRINKING-AGE POPULATION, U.S.A. 1970*

State	Distilled Spirits	Absolute Alcohol	Wine	Absolute Alcohol	Beer	Absolute Alcohol	TOTAL Absolute Alcohol
Alabama	1.59	0.72	0.58	0.09	13.66	0.61	**1.42**
Alaska	4.79	2.16	2.36	0.38	27.22	1.22	**3.76**
Arizona	2.41	1.08	2.03	0.32	31.30	1.41	**2.81**
Arkansas	1.35	0.61	0.86	0.13	16.20	0.73	**1.47**
California	3.12	1.40	4.06	0.65	25.20	1.13	**3.18**
Colorado	2.72	1.22	2.00	0.32	26.96	1.21	**2.75**
Connecticut	3.34	1.50	2.17	0.35	22.81	1.03	**2.88**
Delaware	4.14	1.86	1.38	0.22	26.82	1.21	**3.29**
Florida	3.58	1.61	1.89	0.30	24.86	1.12	**3.03**
Georgia	2.32	1.04	0.89	0.14	18.06	0.81	**1.99**
Hawaii	2.58	1.16	1.61	0.26	25.35	1.14	**2.56**
Idaho	1.72	0.77	0.63	0.10	27.48	1.24	**2.11**
Illinois	3.05	1.37	1.74	0.28	27.72	1.25	**2.90**
Indiana	1.68	0.76	0.77	0.12	22.94	1.03	**1.91**
Iowa	1.56	0.70	0.39	0.06	24.93	1.12	**1.88**
Kansas	1.48	0.67	0.59	0.09	19.52	0.88	**1.64**
Kentucky	1.94	0.87	0.53	0.08	21.38	0.96	**1.91**
Louisiana	2.13	0.96	1.85	0.30	27.60	1.24	**2.50**
Maine	2.36	1.06	0.62	0.10	28.30	1.27	**2.43**
Maryland	3.17	1.43	1.63	0.26	29.89	1.35	**3.04**

*(National Institute of Mental Health, 1972)

State	Distilled Spirits	Absolute Alcohol	Wine	Absolute Alcohol	Beer	Absolute Alcohol	TOTAL Absolute Alcohol
Massachusetts	3.09	1.39	1.92	0.31	26.12	1.18	**2.88**
Michigan	2.44	1.10	1.54	0.25	31.45	1.42	**2.77**
Minnesota	2.65	1.19	1.01	0.16	26.09	1.17	**2.52**
Mississippi	1.62	0.73	0.53	0.08	18.88	0.85	**1.66**
Missouri	2.28	1.03	1.25	0.20	25.68	1.16	**2.39**
Montana	2.35	1.06	0.86	0.14	35.31	1.59	**2.79**
Nebraska	2.33	1.05	0.85	0.14	29.33	1.32	**2.51**
Nevada	7.25	3.26	4.30	0.69	39.51	1.78	**5.73**
New Hampshire	6.44	2.90	2.02	0.32	38.36	1.73	**4.95**
New Jersey	3.15	1.42	2.44	0.39	26.72	1.20	**3.01**
New Mexico	2.26	1.02	2.36	0.38	27.56	1.24	**2.64**
New York	3.26	1.47	2.55	0.41	26.84	1.21	**3.09**
North Carolina	2.09	0.94	1.02	0.16	16.37	0.74	**1.84**
North Dakota	2.39	1.08	0.69	0.11	27.87	1.25	**2.44**
Ohio	1.86	0.84	1.20	0.19	27.81	1.25	**2.28**
Oklahoma	1.91	0.86	0.94	0.15	17.76	0.80	**1.81**
Oregon	2.06	0.93	2.52	0.40	26.81	1.21	**2.54**
Pennsylvania	1.88	0.85	1.24	0.20	28.82	1.30	**2.35**
Rhode Island	2.68	1.21	2.42	0.39	29.23	1.32	**2.92**
South Carolina	2.88	1.30	1.07	0.17	18.25	0.82	**2.29**
South Dakota	2.08	0.94	0.86	0.14	21.35	0.96	**2.04**
Tennessee	1.33	0.60	0.41	0.07	19.91	0.90	**1.57**
Texas	1.74	0.78	1.12	0.18	30.02	1.35	**2.31**
Utah	1.31	0.59	0.79	0.13	17.28	0.78	**1.50**
Vermont	3.96	1.78	2.48	0.40	31.64	1.42	**3.60**
Virginia	2.32	1.04	1.32	0.21	25.44	1.14	**2.39**
Washington	2.46	1.11	2.51	0.40	27.26	1.23	**2.74**
West Virginia	1.57	0.71	0.57	0.09	19.79	0.89	**1.69**
Wisconsin	2.86	1.29	1.40	0.22	39.19	1.76	**3.27**
Wyoming	2.64	1.19	1.01	0.16	29.39	1.32	**2.67**
D.C.	**10.39**	**4.68**	**5.24**	**0.84**	**31.48**	**1.42**	**6.94**
U.S.A.	2.56	1.15	1.84	0.29	25.95	1.17	**2.61**

Appendix III

APPARENT ANNUAL CONSUMPTION, OVER TIME, OF EACH MAJOR BEVERAGE CLASS, AND OF ABSOLUTE ALCOHOL FROM EACH CLASS, IN U.S. GALLONS PER PERSON IN THE DRINKING-AGE POPULATION, U.S.A. 1850-1970*

Year	Distilled Spirits	Absolute Alcohol	Wine	Absolute Alcohol	Beer	Absolute Alcohol	Total
1850	4.17	1.88	0.46	0.08	2.70	0.14	**2.10**
1860	4.79	2.16	0.57	0.10	5.39	0.27	**2.53**
1870	3.40	1 53	0.53	0.10	8.73	0.44	**2.07**
1871-80	2.27	1.02	0.77	0.14	11.26	0.56	**1.72**
1881-90	2.12	0.95	0.76	0.14	17.94	0.90	**1.99**
1891-95	2.12	0.95	0.60	0.11	23.42	1.17	**2.23**
1896-1900	1.72	0.77	0.55	0.10	23.72	1.19	**2.06**
1901-05	2.11	0.95	0.71	0.13	26.20	1.31	**2.39**
1906-10	2.14	0.96	0.92	0.17	29.27	1.47	**2.60**
1911-15	2.09	0.94	0.79	0.14	29.53	1.48	**2.56**
1916-19	1.68	0.76	0.69	0.12	21.63	1.08	**1.96**

PROHIBITION (Figures Unavailable)

Year	Distilled Spirits	Absolute Alcohol	Wine	Absolute Alcohol	Beer	Absolute Alcohol	Total
1934	0.64	0.29	0.36	0.07	13.58	0.61	**0.97**
1935	0.96	0.43	0.50	0.09	15.13	0.68	**1.20**
1936	1.20	0.59	0.64	0.12	17.53	0.79	**1.50**
1937	1.43	0.64	0.71	0.13	18.21	0.82	**1.59**
1938	1.32	0.59	0.70	0.13	16.58	0.75	**1.47**
1939	1.38	0.62	0.79	0.14	16.77	0.75	**1.51**
1940	1.43	0.67	0.01	0.16	16.29	0.73	**1.56**

*(National Institute of Mental Health, 1972)

Year	Distilled Spirits	Absolute Alcohol	Wine	Absolute Alcohol	Beer	Absolute Alcohol	Total
1941	1.58	0.71	1.02	0.18	17.97	0.81	1.70
1942	1.89	0.85	1.11	0.20	20.00	0.90	1.95
1943	1.46	0.66	0.94	0.17	22.26	1.00	1.83
1944	1.00	0.76	0.02	0.17	25.22	1.13	2.06
1945	1.95	0.88	1.13	0.20	25.97	1.17	2.25
1946	2.20	0.99	1.34	0.24	23.75	1.07	2.30
1947	1.69	0.76	0.90	0.16	24.56	1.11	2.03
1948	1.56	0.70	1.11	0.20	23.77	1.07	1.97
1949	1.55	0.70	1.21	0.22	23.48	1.06	1.98
1950	1.72	0.77	1.27	0.23	23.21	1.04	2.04
1951	1.73	0.78	1.13	0.20	22.92	1.03	2.01
1952	1.63	0.73	1.22	0.21	23.20	1.04	1.98
1953	1.70	0.77	1.19	0.20	23.04	1.04	2.01
1954	1.66	0.74	1.21	0.21	22.41	1.01	1.96
1955	1.71	0.77	1.25	0.22	22.39	1.01	2.00
1956	1.31	0.81	1.27	0.22	22.18	1.00	2.03
1957	1.77	0.80	1.26	0.22	21.44	0.97	1.99
1958	1.77	0.80	1.27	0.22	21.35	0.96	1.98
1959	1.86	0.84	1.28	0.22	22.15	1.00	2.06
1960	1.90	0.86	1.32	0.22	21.95	0.99	2.07
1961	1.91	0.86	1.36	0.23	21.47	0.97	2.06
1962	1.99	0.90	1.32	0.22	21.98	0.99	2.11
1963	2.02	0.91	1.37	0.23	22.51	1.01	2.15
1964	2.01	0.95	1.41	0.24	23.08	1.04	2.23
1965	2.21	0.99	1.42	0.24	23.07	1.04	2.27
1966	2.26	1.02	1.40	0.24	23.52	1.06	2.32
1967	2.34	1.05	1.46	0.25	23.81	1.07	2.37
1968	2.44	1.10	1.51	0.26	24.33	1.09	2.45
1969	2.51	1.13	1.62	0.26	24.90	1.12	2.51
1970	2.56	1.15	1.84	0.29	26.95	1.17	2.61

Appendix IV

DRUG AND CHEMICAL BLOOD
LEVEL DATA†

Definition of Blood Levels

THERAPEUTIC BLOOD LEVEL. Fochtman and Winek defined a therapeutic blood level as that concentration of drug present in the blood (its serum or plasma) following therapeutically effective dosage in humans.

TOXIC BLOOD LEVEL. The concentration of drug or chemical present in the blood (its serum or plasma) that is associated with serious toxic symptoms in humans.

LETHAL BLOOD LEVEL. The concentration of drug or chemical present in the blood (its serum or plasma) that has been reported to cause death, or is so far above reported therapeutic or toxic concentrations that one can judge that it might cause death in humans.

Compound	Therapeutic or Normal	Toxic	Lethal
A Acetaminophen .... 1 - 2 mg% (Tylenol)		40 mg%	150 mg%
Acetazolamide .... 1 -1.5 mg% (Diamox)		———	———
Acetohexamide .... 2.1 - 5.6 mg% (Dymelor)		———	———
Acetone .... ———		20 - 30 mg%	55 mg%
Acetylsalicylic acid .... 2 - 10 mg% (Salicylate)		15 - 30 mg%	50 mg%
Aluminum .... 0.013 mg%		———	———

*approximately

†Courtesy of Fisher Scientific Company, Pittsburgh, Pennsylvania, distributor. Compiled by Charles L. Winek, Pittsburgh, Pennsylvania.

264

Compound	Therapeutic or Normal	Toxic	Lethal
Ammonia	50 - 170 mcg%	——	——
Aminophylline .... (Theophylline)	2 - 10 mg%	——	——
Amitriptyline .... (Elavil)	2 - 20 mcg%	40 mcg%	1.0 - 2.0 mg%
Amphetamine	2 - 3 mcg%	——	0.2 mg%
Arsenic	0.0 - 0.002 mg%	0.1 mg%	1.5 mg%
Aventyl .... (Nortriptyline)	12 - 16 mcg%	0.5 mg%	1.3 mg%

B Barbiturates

short acting	0.1 mg%	0.7 mg%	1 mg%
immediate acting	0.1 - 0.5 mg%	1 - 3 mg%	3 mg% & >
phenobarbital	ca. * 1.0 mg%	4 - 6 mg%	8 - 15 mg & >
barbital	ca. 1.0 mg%	6 - 8 mg%	10 mg% & >
Benadryl .... (Diphenhydramine)	0.5 mg%	1 mg%	——
Benemid .... (Probenecid)	10 - 20 mg%	——	——
Benzedrex .... (Propylhexedrine)	——	——	0.2 - 0.3 mg%
Benzene	——	any measurable	0.094 mg%
Beryllium	tissue levels generally used (lung & lymph)	——	——
Boron .... (Boric acid)	0.08 mg%	4 mg%	5 mg%
Bromide	5.0 mg%	50 - 150 mg% (17 mEql)	200 mg%
Brompheniramine .... (Dimetane)	0.8 - 1.5 mcg%	——	——
Butazolidin .... (Phenylbutazone)	ca. 10 mg%	——	——

C
Cadmium	0.01 - 0.02 mcg%	0.005 mg%	——
Caffeine	——	——	10 mg% & >
Carbamazepine .... (Tegretol)	0.2 mg%	0.8 - 1.0 mg%	——
Carbon monoxide	1%	15 - 35%	50%
Carbon tetrachloride	——	2 - 5 mg%	——
Carisoprodol .... (Rela, Soma)	1.0 - 4.0 mg%	——	——
Celontin .... (Methsuximide)	0.25 - 0.75 mg%	——	——
Chloral hydrate .... (Noctec)	1.0 mg%	10 mg%	25 mg%
Chloroform	——	7-25 mg%	39 mg%

Compound	Therapeutic or Normal	Toxic	Lethal
Chlordiazepoxide .... (Librium)	0.1 - 0.3 mg%	0.55 mg%	2 mg%
Chlorpheniramine	———	2 - 3 mg%	———
Chlorpromazine .... (Thorazine)	0.05 mg%	0.1 - 0.2 mg%	0.3 - 1.2 mg%
Chlorpropamide .... (Diabinese)	3.0 - 14.0 mg%	———	———
Chlorprothixine .... (Taractan)	0.004 - 0.03 mg%	———	———
Codeine	2.5 mcg%	———	20 -60 mcg%
Copper	100 - 150 mcg%	540 mcg%	———
Compazine .... (Prochlorperazine)	———	0.1 mg%	———
Cyanide	0.015 mg%	———	0.5 mg% & >
D Darvon .... (Dextropropoxyphene)	5 - 20 mcg%	0.5 - 1 mg%	5.7 mg%
DDT	1.3 mcg%	———	———
Demerol .... (Meperidine)	60 - 65 mcg%	0.5 mg%	ca. 3 mg%
Despramine .... (Norpramin)	.059 - 0.14 mg%	———	1 - 2 mg%
Dextropropoxyphene .... (Darvon)	5 - 20 mcg%	0.5 - 1 mg%	5.7 mg%
Diabinese .... (Chlorpropamide)	3.0 - 14.0 mg%	———	———
Diamox .... (Acetazolamide)	1 - 1.5 mg%	———	———
Diazepam .... (Valium)	0.05 - 0.25 mg%	0.5 - 2.0 mg%	2.0 mg% & >
Dieldrin	0.15 mcg%	———	———
Digitoxin	0.07 - 0.21 mcg%	———	32 mcg%
Digoxin	0.06 - 0.13 mcg%	0.20 - 0.90 mcg%	———
Dilantin .... (Diphenylhydantoin)	0.5 - 2.2 mg%	5 mg%	10 mg% & >
Dilaudid .... (Hydromorphone)	———	———	0.01 - 0.03 mg%
Dimetane .... (Brompheniramine)	0.8 - 1.5 mcg%	———	———
Dinitro-o-Cresol	———	3 - 4 mg%	7.5 mg%
Diphenhydramine .... (Benadryl)	0.5 mg%	1 mg%	———
Diphenylhyantoin .... (Dilantin)	0.5 - 2.2 mg%	5 mg%	10 mg% & >
Divinyl oxide	———	———	70 mg%
Doriden .... (Glutethimide)	0.02 mg%	1 - 8 mg%	3 - 10 mg%

Compound	Therapeutic or Normal	Toxic	Lethal
Doxepin .... ——		——	1.0 mg% & >
(Sinequan)			
Dymelor .... 2.1 - 5.6 mg%		——	——
(Acetohexamide)			
E Elavil .... 5 - 20 mcg%		40 mcg%	1.0 - 2.0 mg%
(Amitriptyline)			
Ethanol .... ——		150 mg%	350 mg% & >
Ethchlorvynol .... ca. 0.5 mg%		2 mg%	15 mg%
(Placidyl)			
Ethinamate .... 0.5 - 1.0 mg%		——	——
(Valmid)			
Ethosuximide .... 2.5 - 7.5 mg%		——	——
(Zarontin)			
Ethyl chloride .... ——		——	40 mg%
Ethyl ether .... 90 - 100 mg%		——	140 - 189 mg%
Ethylene glycol .... ——		150 mg%	200 - 400 mg%
F Fenfluramine .... 10 - 12 mcg%		0.02 - 0.09 mg%	0.6 - 1.5 mg%
(Pondimin)			
Flexin .... 0.3 - 1.3 mg%		——	——
(Zoxazolamine)			
Fluoride .... 0 - 0.05 mg%		——	0.2 mg%
Fluothane .... 0.18 mg%		——	20 mg%
(Halothane)			
Furadantin .... 0.18 mg%		——	——
(Nitrofurantoin)			
G Gantrisin .... 9 - 10 mg%		——	——
(Sulfisoxazole)			
Gold .... 300 - 600 mcg%		——	——
(Sodium aurothiomalate)			
Glutethimide .... 0.02 mg%		1 - 8 mg%	3 - 10 mg%
(Doriden)			
H Halothane .... ——		——	20 mg%
(Fluothane)			
Hydrogen sulfide .... ——		——	0.092 mg%
Hydromorphine .... ——		——	0.01 - 0.03 mg%
(Dilaudid)			
I Imipramine .... 0.005 - 0.016 mg%		> 0.07 mg%	0.2 mg%
(Tofranil)			
Inderal .... 0.0025 - 0.02 mg%		——	0.8 - 1.2 mg%
(Propranolol)			
Isopropanol .... ——		340 mg%	——
Iron .... 50 mg% (RBC)		0.6 mg% (serum)	——

Compound	Therapeutic or Normal	Toxic	Lethal
J Lead	0.005 - 0.13 mg%	0.07 mg%	———
Librium .... (Chlordiazepoxide)	0.1 - 0.3 mg%	0.55 mg%	2 mg%
Lidocaine	0.2 mg%	0.6 mg%	———
Lithium	0.42 - 0.83 mg% (0.6 - 1.2 mEq/l)	1.39 mg% (2.0 mEq/l)	1.39 - 3.47 mg% (2.0 - 5.0 mEq/l)
L.S.D.	———	0.1 - 0.4 mcg%	
M Madribon .... (Sulfadimethoxine)	8 - 10 mg%	———	———
Magnesium	1.5 - 2.5 mg%	———	5 mg%
Manganese	0.015 mg%	0.46 mg%	———
Mellaril .... (Thioridazine)	0.10 - 0.15 mg%	1.0 mg%	2 - 8 mg%
Meperidine .... (Demerol)	60 - 65 mcg%	0.5 mg%	ca. 3 mg%
Meprobamate	1 mg%	10 mg%	20 mg%
Mercury	0.006 - 0.012 mg%	———	
Methadone	48 - 86 mcg%	0.2 mg%	0.4 mg% & >
Methamphetamine	———	0.5 mg%	4 mg%
Methanol	———	20 mg%	89 mg% & >
Methapyrilene	0.2 - 0.4 mg%	3 - 5 mg%	5 mg% & >
Methaqualone .... (Quaalude)	0.5 mg%	1 - 3 mg%	3 mg% & >
Methsuximide .... (Celontin)	0.25 - 0.75 mg%	———	———
Methylene chloride	———	———	28 mg%
Methylenedioxyamphetamine .. (MDA)	———	———	0.4 - 1.0 mg%
Methyprylon .... (Noludar)	1.0 mg%	3 - 6 mg%	10 mg%
Milontin .... (Phensuximide)	1 - 1.9 mg%	———	———
Morphine	0.01 mg%	———	0.005 - 0.4 mg% (free morphine from heroin
Mysoline .... (Primidone)	1.0 mg%	5 - 8 mg%	ca 10 mg%
N Nickel	0.041 mg%	———	———
Nicotine	———	1 mg%	0.5 - 5.2 mg%
Nitrofurantoin .... (Furadantin)	0.18 mg%	-———	———
Noctec .... (Chloral hydrate)	1.0 mg%	10 mg%	25 mg%
Noludar .... (Methyprylon)	1.0 mg%	3 - 6 mg%	10 mg%

Compound	Therapeutic or Normal	Toxic	Lethal
Norpramin .... .059 - 0.14 mg% (Desipramine)		——	1 - 2 mg%
Nortriptyline .... 12 - 16 mcg% (Aventyl)		0.5 mg%	1.3 mg%
O Orinase .... 5.3 - 9.6 mg% (Tolbutamide)		——	——
Orphenadrine .... ——		0.2 mg%	0.4 - 0.8 mg%
Oxalate .... 0.2 mg%		——	1.0 mg%
P Papaverine .... ——		——	——
Para-methoxyamphetamine ... 0.1 mg% (PMA)		——	0.2 - 0.4 mg%
Paraldehyde .... ca. 5.0 mg%		20 - 40 mg%	50 mg%
Pentazocine .... 0.014 - 0.016 mg% (Talwin)		0.2 - 0.5 mg%	1 - 2 mg%
Perphenazine .... —— (Trilafon)		0.1 mg%	——
Phencyclidine .... ——		——	0.1 mg%
Phenmetrazine .... ——		——	0.4 mg%
Phensuximide .... 1 - 1.9 mg% (Milontin)		——	——
Phenylbutazone .... ca. 10 mg% (Butazolidin)		——	——
Phosphorus .... tissue levels usually used			
Placidyl .... ca. 0.5 mg% (Ethchlorvynol)		2 mg%	15 mg%
Primidone .... 1.0 mg% (Mysoline)		5 - 8 mg%	ca. 10 mg%
Probenecid .... 10 - 20 mg% (Benemid)		——	——
Procainamide .... 0.6 mg%		1 mg%	——
Prochlorperazine .... —— (Compazine)		0.1 mg%	——
Promazine .... —— (Sparine)		0.1 mg%	——
Propoxyphene .... 5 - 20 mcg%		0.5 - 2 mg%	5.7 mg%
Propranolol .... 0.0025 - 0.02 mg% (Inderal)		——	0.8 - 1.2 mg%
Propylhexedrine .... —— (Benzedrex)		——	0.2- 0.3 mg%
Q Quaalude .... 0.5 mg% (Methaqualone)		1 - 3 mg%	3 mg% & >
Quinidine .... 0.03 - 0.6 mg%		ca. 1.0 mg%	3 - 5 mg%
Quinine .... ——		——	1.2 mg>

Compound	Therapeutic or Normal	Toxic	Lethal
R Rela, Soma .... 1.0 - 4.0 mg%		——	——
(Carisoprodol)			
S Salicylate .... 2 - 10 mg%		15 - 30 mg%	50 mg%
(acetylsalicylic acid)			
Sinequan .... ——		——	1.0 mg% & >
(Doxepin)			
Sodium aurothiomalate .... 300 - 600 mcg%		——	——
(Gold)			
Soma, Rela .... 1.0 - 4.0 mg%		——	——
(Carisoprodol)			
Sparine .... ——		0.1 mg%	——
(Promazine)			
Sulfadiazine .... 8 - 15 mg%		——	——
Sulfadimethoxine .... 8 - 10 mg%		——	——
(Madribon)			
Sulfaguanidine .... 3 - 5 mg%		——	——
Sulfanilamide .... 10 - 15 mg%		——	——
Sulfisoxazole .... 9 - 10 mg%		——	——
(Gantrisin)			
Strychnine .... ——		0.2 ,mg%	0.9 - 1.2 mg%
T Talwin .... 0.014 - 0.016 mg%		0.2 - 0.5 mg%	1 - 2 mg%
(Pentazocine)			
Taractan .... 0.004 - 0.03 mg%		——	——
(Chlorprothixine)			
Tegretol .... 0.2 mg%		0.8 - 1.0 mg%	——
(Carbamazepine)			
Theophylline .... 2 - 10 mg%		——	——
(Aminophylline)			
Thioridazine .... 0.10 - 0.15 mg%		1.0 mg%	2 - 8 mg%
(Mellaril)			
Thorazine .... 0.05 mg%		0.1 - 0.2 mg%	0.3 - 1.2 mg%
(Chlorpromazine)			
Tigan .... 0.1 - 0.2 mg%		——	——
(Trimethobenzamide)			
Tin .... 0.012 mg%		——	——
Tofranil .... 0.005 - 0.016 mg%		> 0.07 mg%	0.2 mg%
(Imipramine)			
Tolbutamide .... 5.3 - 9.6 mg%		——	——
(Orinase)			
Toluene .... ——		——	1.0 mg%
Tribromoethanol .... ——		——	9 mg%
Trichloroethane .... ——		——	10 - 100 mg%
Trilafon .... ——		——	0.1 mg%
(Perphenazine)			

Compound	Therapeutic or Normal	Toxic	Lethal
Trimethobenzamide .... 0.1 - 0.2 mg% (Tigan)		———	———
Tylenol .... 1 - 2 mg% (Acetaminophen)		40 mg%	150 mg%
U Uric Acid .... 3-7 mg%		———	———
V Valmid .... 0.5 - 1.0 mg% (Ethinamate)		———	———
Valium .... 0.05 - 0.25 mg% (Diazepam)		0.5 - 2.0 mg%	2.0 mg% & >
W Warfarin .... 0.1 - 1.0 mg%		———	———
Z Zarontin .... 2.5 - 7.5 mg% (Ethosuximide)		———	———
Zinc .... 68 - 136 mcg%		———	———
Zoxavolamine .... 0.3 - 1.3 mg% (Flexin)		———	———

Appendix V

MINIMUM LETHAL DOSE OF SOME
REPRESENTATIVE VOLATILE
HYDROCARBONS

Hydrocarbon	*Minimum Lethal Dose*
Acetone	100 ml
Amyl acetate	50 gm
Benzene	15 ml
Carbon disulfide	10 ml
Carbon tetrachloride	5 ml
Naphthol	2 gm
Nitrobenzene	2 ml
Ether	25 ml
Ethyl acetate	100 ml
Toluene	50 gm
Trichloroethylene	5 ml
Turpentine	30 ml
Xylene	50 gm

REFERENCES

Alexander, J.F. and R. Rosario. 1971. A case of mercury poisoning: Acrodynia in a child of 8. *Can Med Assoc J, 104 (10)*:929-930.

Allen, T.H. and R.W. Allard. 1961. *Fundamental Parameters Influencing the Accumulation and Elimination of Carbon Monoxide by Adult Human Beings.* Report No. 261. U.S. Army Medical Research and Nutrition Laboratory, Denver, Colorado.

Arena, J.M. 1966. The treatment of poisoning. *Clin Symp, 18 (1)*:3-31.

Back, K.C. and E.W. Van Stee. 1977. Toxicology of haloalkane propellants and fire extinguishants. *Ann Rev Pharmacol Toxicol, 17*:83-95.

Bank, W.J., D.E. Pleasure, K. Suzuki, M. Nigro, and R. Katz 1972. Thallium poisoning. *Arch Neurol, 26*:456-464.

Bartholomew, A.A. 1967. Alcoholism and driving efficiency. *Med J Aust, 2 (16)*:721-724.

Berman, E. 1966. The biochemistry of lead: Review of the body distribution and methods of lead determination. *Clin Pediatr, 5 (5)*:287-291.

Bird, D. 1978. 2 of 5 murder charges dismissed by judge in the Jascalevich case. *New York Times,* Wednesday, 2 August 1978. pp. Al, A15.

Blum, K., M.G. Hamilton, J.E. Wallace. 1977. Alcohol and opiates: A review of common neurochemical and behavioral mechanisms. *In* Blum, K. (Ed.): *Alcohol and Opiates.* Academic Press, New York, pp. 203-236.

Blume, P. and D.J. Lakatua. 1973. Effect of microbial contamination of the blood sample in the determination of ethanol levels in serum. *Am J Clin Pathol, 60*:700-702.

Castro, A. and H. Malkus. 1977. Radioimmunoassays of drugs of abuse in humans: A review. *Res Commun Chem Pathol Pharmacol, 16 (2)*:291-309.

Chafetz, M. 1972. Fact and Myth in Alcoholism. *Ann N.Y. Acad Sci, 197*:8-10.

Chafetz, M. 1972. *Alcohol and Alcoholism.* National Institute of Mental Health. DHEW Publ. No. (HSM) 72-9127. U.S. Government Printing Office, Washington, D.C. 42 pp.

Chisolm, J.J. 1970. Poisoning due to heavy metals. *Pediatr Clin North Am, 17 (3)*:591-615.

Choulis, N.H. 1976. *Identification Procedures of Drugs of Abuse.* European Press, Ghent.

Christensen, H.E. (Ed.). 1973. *Toxic Substances List,* 1973 ed., HSM 73-11020. Public Health Service, Rockville, Maryland.

Citation. 1973. Alcoholic released from hospital. *Citation, 28(3):*40-41.

Clinical Toxicology. 1972. Special communication: Thallium poisoning. *Clin Toxicol, 5(1):*89-93.

Coburn, R.F. (Ed.) 1970. Biological effects of carbon monoxide. *Ann NY Acad Sci, 174:*1-430.

Coe, J.I. 1974. Postmortem chemistry: Practical considerations and a review of the literature. *J Forensic Sci, 19 (1):*13-32.

Comstock, E.G. 1968. The treatment of poisoning: A program for the medical curriculum. *Clinical Toxicology, 1(1):*49-56.

Cook, W.A. 1966. Noxious gases. In Clark, G.L. (Ed.). *Encyclopedia of Chemistry,* 2nd ed. Reinhold, New York, pp. 703-707.

Cumings, J.N. 1967. Trace metals in the brain and their importance in human disease. *Chem Weekbl, 63 (42):*473-479.

Cumont, G. 1972. Utilisation et consommation du mercure en France. Ebauche des problèmes sanitaires qui en découlant. *Rec Med Vet, 148:* 427-442.

Curry, A.S. 1972. *Advances in Forensic and Clinical Toxicology.* The Chemical Rubber Co., Cleveland, Ohio.

Davis, J.H. 1974. Carbon monoxide, alcohol, and drugs in fatal automibile accidents in Dade County, Florida. *Clin Toxicol, 7 (6):*597-613.

Department of the Army. 1966. *Chemical Biological, and Nuclear Defense.* Field Manual No. 21-40. U.S. Government Printing Office, Washington, D.C.

Department of the Army. 1968. *Civil Disturbances and Disasters.* Field Manual No. 19-15. U.S. Government Printing Office, Washington, D.C.

Diem, K. (Ed.). 1962. *Documenta Geigy Scientific Tables,* 6th ed. Geigy Pharmaceuticals, Ardsley, New York.

DiMaio, V.J.M. and J.C. Garriott. 1978. Four deaths resulting from abuse of nitrous oxide. *J Forensic Sci, 23 (1):*169-172.

D'Itri, P.A. and F.M. D'Itri. 1977. *Mercury Cotamination: A Human Tragedy.* Wiley & Sons, New York.

D'Itri, P.A. and F.M. D'Itri. 1978. Mercury contamination: A human tragedy. *Environmental Management, 2 (1):*3-6.

Dominquez, A.M. 1962. Problems of carbon monoxide in fires. *J Forensic Sci, 7 (4):*379-393.

Done, A.K. 1961. Pharmacology of systemic antidotes. *Clin Pharmacol Ther, 2 (6):*750-793.

Done, A. 1968. *Short and Long-Term Effects of Acute Poisoning.* U.S. Public Health Service Publication No. 1791. U.S. Government Printing Office, Washington, D.C., p.p. 155-163.

Drug Enforcement Administration. 1979. *Instrumental Applications in Forensic Drug Chemistry.* United States Department of Justice. Drug

Enforcement Administration. Office of Science and Technology. Forensic Sciences Division. Special Testing and Research Laboratory. Proceedings of the International Symposium. May 29-30, 1978. Washington, D.C.

Duncan, C.W. 1978. *Drug Abuse in the Military.* Supplement to the Air Force Policy Letter for Commanders, No. 10-1978. U.S. Air Force, Washington, D.C., AFRP 190-2, 9-15.

Eckert, W.D. and T.T. Noguchi, (Eds.) 1973. *Alcohol and Alcoholism. The Medical, Legal and Law Enforcement Aspects.* International Reference Organization in Forensic Medicine and Sciences (INFORM), Witchita, Kansas.

Eckert, W.G. and T.T. Noguchi (Eds.). 1973. *A Bibliography of Classic and Current References on Alcohol and Alcoholism,* vol. 1, *Alcohol.* International Reference Organization in Forensic Medicine and Sciences (INFORM), Witchita, Kansas.

Edds, G.T. 1950. *BAL, Antidote for Arsenic and Other Metals.* Proceedings Book Am Vet Med Assoc 87th Ann Meet, Aug. 1950, pp. 149-153.

Edgewood Arsenal. 1967. *Characteristics of Riot Control Agent CS.* Edgewood Arsenal Special Publication (EASP) 600-1. Department of Army, Army Chemical Center, Maryland.

Faivre, M.I. 1978. *Suicide. A Cry for Help.* Pamphlet Publications, Div. RMA. Cincinnati, Ohio.

Finck, P.A. 1966. Exposure to carbon monoxide. Review of the literature and 567 autopsies. *Milit Med, 131(12):*1513-1539.

Finkle, B.S. and K.L. McCloskey. 1978. The forensic toxicology of cocaine (1971-1976). *J Forensic Sci, 23 (1):*173-189.

Fisher, R.S. and H.C. Freimuth. 1956. Common poisoning and their management. *Med Clin North Am, 40 (5):*1489-1501.

Foreman, H. 1962. Toxicology: Inorganic. *Annu Rev Pharmacol, 2:*341-362.

Foulger, J.H. 1959. *Chemicals, Drugs, and Health.* Charles C Thomas Publisher, Springfield.

Fox, R.H. and C.L. Cunningham. 1973. *Crime Scene Search and Physical Evidence Handbook.* U.S. Department of Justice, Law Enforcement Assistance Administration, U.S. Government Printing Office, Washington, D.C.

Francke, D. 1974. Adverse drug reactions in perspective. *Drug Intelligence and Clinical Pharmacy,* 8.

Freireich, A.W., J.H. Bidanset, and L. Lukash. 1975. Alcohol levels in intracranial blood clots. *J Forensic Sci, 20(1):*83-85.

Furneaux, R. 1957. *The Medical Murderer.* Abelarde-Schuman, New York.

Gaddum, J.H. 1953. Bioassays and mathematics. *Pharmacol Rev, 5:*87-134.

Geldmacher v. Mallinckrodt, M., A. Zober, J. Dumbach, J.H. Geldmacher, L. Lautenbach, G. Machbert, G. Reinhardt, G. Schaidt, B. Schellmann, W. Schütz, H.-B. Wuermeling, and P. Zink. 1976. Deaths resulting from the combined effect of alcohol and drugs. *Z Rechtsmed, 78(2)*:97-129.

German Commission. 1976. Breath alcohol testing cannot replace blood alcohol determination. *JAMA, 226 (9)*:129.

Gleason, M.N., R.E. Gosselin, H.C. Hodge, and R.P. Smith. 1969. Clinical toxicology of commercial products, 3rd ed. Williams & Wilkins, Baltimore, Maryland.

Gold, M., E. Tassoni, and M. Etzl. 1973. Comparison of glutethimide concentration in the serum and cerebrospinal fluid of humans in drug overdose. *Clin Chem, 19*:1158-1161.

Goldbaum, L.R. and M.A. Williams. 1968. Identification and determination of micrograms of morphine in biological samples. *J Forensic Sci, 13*:253.

Goldsmith, J.R. and S.I. Cohen. 1969. Epidemiological bases for possible air quality criteria for carbon monoxide. *J Air Pollut Control Assoc,* 19 *(9)*:704-713.

Goodwin, D.W. 1973. Alcohol in suicide and homicide. *Q J Stud Alcohol, 34*:144-156.

Gouveia, W.A., G. Tognoni, and E. van der Kleijn (Eds.) 1976. *Clinical Pharmacy and Clinical Pharmacology.* North-Holland Publishing Co., New York.

Haggerty, R.J. 1975. Common Accidental Poisoning. In *Textbook of Medicine.* Edited by P.B. Beeson and W. McDermott. Saunders, Philadelphia. Vol. 1. pp. 55-57.

Harris, V.G. 1966. In pursuit of more knowledge about accidental poisoning. In: *Safety in the Use of Home Medicines.* The Proprietary Association, Washington, D.C., pp. 61-75.

Hartroft, W.S. 1967. Editor. *Alcohol, Metabolism and Liver Disease.* A Nutrition Society Symposium. Federation Proceedings. *26*:1432-14881.

Hayes, W.J. 1963. *Clinical Handbook on Economic Poisons.* U.S. Department of Health, Education and Welfare, Public Health Service Report No. 476. Communicable Disease Center, Atlanta, Georgia.

Hayes, W.J. 1975. *Toxicology of Pesticides.* William & Wilkins, Baltimore, Maryland.

Herron, C.R. and C. Habermann. 1978. Cold turkey at the White House. *New York Times,* Sunday, 30 July 1978, p. E4.

Hilderbrand, D.C. and D.H. White. 1974. Trace-element analysis in hair: An evaluation. *Clin Chem, 20 (2)*:148-151.

Himwich, H.E. 1957. The physiology of alcohol. *JAMA, 163*:545-549.

Hine, C.H., F.B. Hall, and H.W. Turkel. 1968. Forensic Toxicology for the practicing physician. *Clin Toxicol 1(1)*:71-80.

Hirsch, C., J. Valentour, and L. Adelson. 1973. Unexpected ethanol in drug-intoxicated persons. *Postgrad Med, 54*:53-57.

Hodge, H.C. and J.H. Sterner. 1949. Tabulation of toxicity classes. *AIHA Q, 10*:93-96.

Hoftreuter, D.H., E.J. Catcott, and C. Xintaras. Carboxyhemoglobin in men exposed to carbon monoxide. *Arch Environ Health, 4*:81-85.

Holland, J., M.J. Massie, and C. Grant. 1975. Drugs ingested in suicide attemps and fatal outcome. *NY State J Med, 75 (13)*:2343-2348.

International Association of Chiefs of Police. 1977. *The Police Chief, April:* p. 10.

Irvine, A. and H. Johnson. 1974. R. v. Young—Murder by thallium. *Med Leg J, 42 (3)*:76-90.

Jackson, G.W. and A. Richman. 1973. Alcohol use among narcotic addicts. *Alcohol Health and Research World. 1(1)*:25 28.

Johnston, E.H., L.R. Goldbaum, and R.L. Whelton. 1969. Investigation of sudden deaths in addicts. *Med Ann DC, 38*:375-380.

Joint Committee on New York Drug Law Evaluation. 1977. *Nation's Toughest Drug Law—Evaluating the New York Experience—Final Report.* GPO Stock No. 027-000-00648-5, U.S. Government Printing Office, Washington, D.C.

Joint Committee on New York Drug Law Evaluation. 1978A. *Staff Working Papers of the Drug Evaluation Project—A Companion Volume to the Final Report of the Joint Committee on New York Drug Law Evaluation.* GPO Stock No. 027-000-00647-7. U.S. Government Printing Office, Washington, D.C.

Joint Committee on New York Drug Law Evaluation. *Nation's Toughest Drug Law—Evaluating the New York Experience—Executive Summary.* GPO Stock No. 027-000-00651-5. U.S. Government Printing Office, Washington, D.C.

Kalman, S.M. (Ed.). 1971. Riot control agents. Pharmacology Society Symposium. *Fed Proc, 30 (1)*:84-99.

Keiper, C.G. 1972. *Effects of Moderate Blood Alcohol Levels on Driver Alertness.* U.S. Department of Health, Education and Welfare Publication No. (HSM) 72-10017. U.S. Government Printing Office, Washington, D.C.

Keil, S.W. 1966. *Seminar on Poisoning.* American Registry of Pathology, M 14165. Armed Forces Institute of Pathology. Washington, D.C.

Kinsey, B.A. 1966. The problem and the approach: Background and summary of research on the problem of female alcoholism. In Kinsey, B. *The Female Alcoholic: A Social Psychological Study.* Charles C Thomas, Publisher, Springfield, pp. 3-14.

Koch-Weser, J. 1974. Fatal reactions to drug therapy. *N Engl J Med, 291 (6)*.

Lacefield, D.J. 1975. Alcohol continues to play a big part in plane crashes.

*JAMA, 233 (5):*405.

Laurell, H. 1977. Effects of small doses of alcohol on driver performance in emergency traffic situations. *Accident Analysis and Prevention, 9:* 191-201.

Lee, R.V. 1972. Drugs: the stampede into hysteria. *Clin Toxicol, 5:*88-87.

Leonard. 1968. Medical evaluation of CN in the form of Chemical Mace®. Director of Public Health, Berkeley, California.

Leslie, A.C.D. and H. Smith. 1978. Self-poisoning by the abuse of arsenic containing tonics. *Med Sci Law, 18 (3):*159-162.

Loomis, T.A. 1968. *Essentials of Toxicology.* Lea & Febiger, Philadelphia.

Loomis, T.A. 1974. Blood alcohol in automobile drivers. *Q J Stud Alcohol, 35 (2):*458-472.

MacDonald, J.D. 1978. Coppolino revisited. In Garfield, B. (Ed.). *I Witness.* Times Books, New York, pp. 294-300.

McGuire, F.L. and others. 1976. A comparison of suicide and nonsuicide deaths involving psychotropic drugs in four major U.S. cities. *Am J Public Health, 66 (11):*1058-1061.

McNamarr, B.P. 1944. *Thallium Poisoning: A Review of the Literature.* Medical Division Report No. 15, Publication Control No. 5035-15. Army Service Forces. Office of the Chief, Chemical Warfare Service. Edgewood Arsenal, Maryland.

Mason, M.F. and K.M. Dubowski. 1976. Breath-alcohol analysis: Uses, methods, and some forensic problems—Review and opinion. *J Forensic Sci, 21:*9-41.

Matthew, H. and A.A.H. Lawson. 1975. *Treatment of Common Poisonings,* 3rd ed. Churchill Livingstone, New York.

Mayron, L.W., E. Kaplan, S. Alling. 1974. Drug-abuse and control populations differentiated by a laboratory profile. *Clin Chem 20:*172-176.

Menninger, K. 1938. Alcohol addiction. In Menninger, K. (Ed.). *Man Against Himself.* Harcourt, Brace, New York, pp. 140-161.

Ministry of Labour. 1955. Carbon monoxide. In *Methods for the Detection of Toxic Substances in Air.* Booklet No. 7. Her Majesty's Stationery Office, London.

Morrell, G. 1978. Clinical forum: Arsenic poisoning. *Laboratory Management, 16 (5):*54-55.

Morselli, P.L., S. Garattini, and S.N. Cohen (Eds.). 1974. *Drug Interactions.* Raven Press, New York.

National Clearinghouse for Alcohol Information. 1974. *Subject Area: Bibliography on Suicide and Alcohol.* No. 8. Department of Health, Education and Welfare Publication No. (ADM) 75-172. National Institute on Alcohol Abuse and Alcoholism, Rockville, Maryland. Ross Abstract.

National Clearinghouse for Alcohol Information. 1976. *Physiologic Concomitants of Alcohol Use and Abuse.* Grouped interest guide No. 9-5.

U.S. Department of Health, Education and Welfare Publication No. (ADM) 76-272. National Institute on Alcohol Abuse and Alcoholism, Rockville, Maryland.

National Clearinghouse for Alcohol Information. 1978. IFS No. 51. National Institute on Alcohol Abuse and Alcoholism, Rockville, Maryland.

National Dairy Council. 1977. Diet-Drug Interactions. An interpretive review of recent nutrition research. *Dairy Council Digest, 48(2).* (ISSN 0011-5568).

National Institute of Mental Health. 1972. *Alcohol and Alcoholism. Problems, Programs, and Progress,* revised. U.S. Department of Health, Education and Welfare Publication No. (HSM) 72-9127. National Institute on Alcohol Abuse and Alcoholism. U.S. Government Printing Office. Washington, D.C.

Notional Institute on Alcohol Abuse and Alcoholism. 1971. *Alcohol. Some Questions and Answers.* U.S. Department of Health Education and Welfare Publication No. (HSM) 71-9048. U.S. Government Printing Office, Rockville, Maryland.

National Research Council. 1977. *Arsenic.* Committee on medical and biologic effects of environmental pollutants, National Academy of Sciences, Washington, D.C.

New York Times. 1978. Two die of car fumes. Monday, 24 July 1978, pp. A3 and B3.

Paget, G.E. (Ed.). 1970. *Methods in Toxicology.* Blackwell, Oxford.

Palmes, E.D. 1976. Letter to the editor. *Clin Toxicol, 9 (5):723-730.*

Pankow, D., W. Ponsold, and H. Fritz. 1974. Combined effects of carbon monoxide and ethanol. *Arch Toxicol, 32 (4):331-340.*

Penneys, N.S. 1971. Contact dermatitis to chloroacetophenone. *Fed Proc, 30 (1):96-99.*

The Proprietary Association. 1966. *Safety in the Use of Home Medicines.* Proceedings of the Committee on Scientific Development. Research and Scientific Development Conference. The Proprietary Association, Washington, D.C.

Public Health Service. 1970. *Smoking and Health Bulletin.* U.S. Department of Health, Education and Welfare, U.S. Government Printing Office, Washington, D.C.

Public Health Service. 1973. *Poisoning and Intoxication by Trace Elements in Children.* U.S. Department of Health, Education and Welfare Publication No. (HSM) 73-10005. U.S. Government Printing Office, Washington, D.C.

Reddemann, H. and P. Amendt. 1968. Accidental poisoning in childhood. *Arch Kinderheilkd, 177:284-295.*

Reich, G.A., J.H. Davis, and J.E. Davies. 1968. Pesticide poisoning in south Florida. *Arch Environ Health, 17:768-775.*

Reid, E. 1976. *Assay of Drugs and Other Trace Compounds in Biological*

Fluids. North-Holland Publishing Co., London.

Roche Medical Image and Commentary. 1970. CO and cardiac disease. Roche Image and Commentary, 12 (5):6-8.

Rocky Mountain News. 1976. British doctors urged to watch for child-poisoning. *Rocky Mountain News* (Denver, Colorado), Saturday, 3 April, 1976.

Ronaghan, J.T. 1972. *Pharmacodynamics.* U.S. Air Force Academy. Colorado Springs, Colorado.

Rowan, R. and F. Coleman. 1962. Carbon monoxide poisoning. Review of the literature and presentation of a case. *J Forensic Sci, 7 (1):*103-130.

Rushing, W.A. 1969. Suicide and the interaction of alcoholism (liver cirrhosis) with the social situation. *Q J Stud Alcohol, 30 (1A):*93-103.

Rydberg, U. 1977. Experimentally induced alcoholic hangover. In Idestrom, C.-M. (Ed.). *Recent advances in the study of alcoholism.* Excerpta Medica, Amsterdam, pp. 33-40.

Saric, M., S. Lucic-Palaic, and R.J.M. Horton. 1977. Chronic non-specific lung disease and alcohol consumption. *Environ Res, 14:*14-21.

Scherz, R.G. 1970. Prevention of childhood poisoning. *Pediatr Clin North Am, 17 (3):*713-727.

Schmidt, C.W., J.W. Shaffer, and W.G. Towns. 1973. *Importance of Human Factors in Vehicular Accidents.* Conference paper in Am Publ Health Adm Meet, Nov. 1973. Baltimore City Hospitals, Department of Psychiatry, Baltimore, Maryland.

Schmidt, R. and C.G. Wilber. 1978. Mercury and lead content of human body tissues from a selected population. *Med Sci Law, 18 (3):*155-158.

Schoene, D., S.T. Waesser, and H. Polster. 1970. The pathological picture of acrodynia. *Kinderaerztl Prax, 38 (9):*390-397.

Schuckit, M. 1972. The alcoholic woman: A literature review. *Psychiatry Med, 3 (1):*37-43.

Secretary of Health, Education and Welfare. 1971. *First Report to the U.S. Congress on Alcohol and Health.* U.S. Department of Health, Education and Welfare, Public Health Service Publication No. (HSM) 76-359. National Institute on Alcohol Abuse and Alcoholism, Rockville, Maryland. Reprinted in 1976.

Seixas, F.A. and S. Eggleston (Eds.). 1976. Work in progress on alcoholism. *Ann NY Acad Sci, 273:*1-664.

Severo, R. 1978. F.T.C. rules urged for funeral industry. *New York Times,* 19 June 1978, pp. A1, A14.

Simon, F.A. and L.K. Pickering. 1976. Acute yellow phosphorus poisoning. "Smoking stool syndrome." *JAMA, 235 (13):*1343-1344.

Simpson, K. (Ed.). 1967. *Modern Trends in Forensic Medicine,* 2nd ed. Butterworths, London.

Solarz, A. 1975. Medical conclusions from the clinical tests of drunken drivers with high alcohol levels. In Isroelstam, S. and S. Lambert (Eds.).

Alcohol, Drugs, and Traffic Safety. Addiction Research Foundation, Toronto, Canada, pp. 389-393.

Spitz, W.U. and R.S. Fisher. 1973. *Medicolegal Investigation of Death.* Charles C Thomas Publisher, Springfield.

Stewart, R., J.E. Baretta, H.C. Dodd, and A.A. Herrman. 1973. Experimental human exposure to high concentrations of carbon monoxide. *Arch Environ Health, 26 (1):*1-7.

Stockton, W. 1978. Dual addiction. *New York Times Magazine,* Sunday, 6 August 1978, section 6, pp. 10-11, 36-41.

Sullivan, R. 1978. An inquiry ordered on claims of overdrugging mental patients. *New York Times.* Tuesday, 18 July 1978. p. B17.

Swearingen, T.F. 1966. *Tear Gas Munitions.* Charles C Thomas, Publisher, Springfield.

Taylor, R.B. 1977. Dr. *Taylor's Self-Help Medical Guide.* Arlington House, New Rochelle, New York.

Temkov, I., K. Kirov, A. Jablenski, and I. Samurkov. 1976. Toxic psychoses from psychostimulant drugs. *Structure and Functions of the Brain. 1:* 333-340.

Theodore, J., R.D. O'Donnell, and K.C. Back. 1971. *Toxicological Evaluation of Carbon Monoxide in Humans and Other Mammalian Species.* Technical Report 71-6. Aerospace Medical Research Laboratory. Wright-Patterson Air Force Base, Dayton, Ohio.

The Toxicology Newsletter. 1977. *The Toxicology Newsletter, 3 (5).*

Truhaut, R. 1958. Thallium poisoning. *Anna Med Leg Criminol, 38:*189-239.

Ulmer, D.D. 1973. Metals—From privation to pollution. *Fed Proc, 32 (7):* 1758-1762.

Underwood Ground, K.E. 1975. Impaired pilot performance; Drugs and alcohol. *Aviation, Space, and Environmental Medicine, 46 (10):*1284-1288.

Usdin, E. and D.H. Efron. 1972. *Psychotropic Drugs and Related Compounds,* 2nd ed. U.S. Department of Health, Education and Welfare Publication No. (HSM) 72-9074. U.S. Government Printing Office, Washington, D.C.

Waldron, H.A. and D. Stofen. 1974. *Subclinical Lead Poisoning.* Academic Press, New York.

Wallace, J.E., H.E. Hamilton, J.A. Riloff. 1974. Spectrophotometric determination of ethchlorvynol in biological specimens. *Clin Chem, 159:*159-162.

Watanabe, T. 1968. *Atlas of Legal Medicine.* Lippincott, Philadelphia.

Wawschinek, O., W. Bayer, and B. Poletta. 1968. Extraktionsphotometrische Thalliumbestimmung in biologischem Material. *Mikrochim Acta 1:*201-204.

Weinraub, B. 1978. A fog and a furor over G. I. drug abuse. *New York*

Times, Sunday, 30 July 1978. p. E4.

Weiss, B. and V.G. Laties (Eds.). 1975. *Behavioral Toxicology.* Plenum Press, New York.

Wells, H.J. 1968. *Forensic Science.* Sweet and Maxwell, London.

Wells, H.J. 1974. *Scotland Yard Scientist.* Taplingen, New York.

Weston, J.T. (Ed.). 1976. *Newsletter.* Office of the Medical Investigator. Albuquerque, New Mexico, *3 (10)*:8; 1977:4 (6).

Wilber, C.G. 1966. Nerve gases. In Clark, G.L. (Ed.). *Encyclopedia of Chemistry,* 2nd ed. Reinhold, New York, pp. 679-681.

Wilber, C.G. 1974. *Forensic Biology for the Law Enforcement Officer.* Charles C Thomas, Publisher, Springfield.

Wilber, C.G. 1978. *Medicolegal Investigation of the President John F. Kennedy Murder.* Charles C Thomas, Publisher, Springfield.

Wilber, C.G. 1978. Chemical trauma from pesticides. Part 1. *Trauma, 20(2)*:5-57; Part 2. *Ibid. 20(3)*9-101; Part 3. 1979, *20(5)*:61-87.

Witter, R.F. 1963. Measurement of blood cholinesterase. *Arch Environ Health, 6*:537-563.

Wolstenholme, G. and R. Porter (Eds.). 1967. *Drug Responses in Man.* Little, Brown and Company, Boston.

Zink, P. and G. Reinhardt. 1976. Die Berechnung der Tatzeit-BAK zur Beurteilung der Schuldfaehigkeit. *Blutalkohl, 13*:327-339.

INDEX

A

Accidental deaths, 40
Accidental poisonings, xii, 26-29
Acetaminophen, 236-237
Achilles' heel of murder, 5
Acrodynia, 185-186
Action of poisons, 36
Activated charcoal, x
Acute poisoning, 23
Acute toxic psychosis, 77-78
Addiction, 65-67
Administrative law, xiv
Adverse reactions to drugs, 94
Age, 16
Alcohol, 15, 19, 42, 71, 106-127
  analyses, 43
  and behavior, 110
  and brain, 111-112
  or carbon monoxide, 117-118
  and heart, 111
  hypersensitivity, Orientals', 251-252
  and life expectancy, 112
  plus narcotics abuse, 116-117
  in New Mexico, 123-127
  and vision, 114-115
  poisoning, 21
  and race, 250
  related disorders, 258-259
  samples, 43-44
  and traffic fatalities, 112
Alcoholism, 106-127
Alkaloidal poisons, 19
Alkaloids, 19
American Academy of Forensic Sciences, 52
Analytical techniques, 55
Anorexia, 37
Anoxia, 18
Anticholinesterase poisoning, 224

Antidote kit, xi
Antidotes, 13, 193-196
Armed Forces, 72-73
Arsenic, 195
  content, human bodies, 203-204
  poisoning, 198-202
  polyneuritis, 204
Art of the poisoner, 3
Asphyxiants, 128
Aspirin, ix, 16
Atmospheric conditions, 32
Automobile air conditioners, 140-141
Autopsy, vii, ix, 26

B

Bacharach Instrument Company, 134
BAL 195-196
Barbiturates, 85-87
Barometric pressure, 32
Beer consumption, 122
Bernard, Claude, 132
Beverages, alcoholic, 109
Bile, 25, 26
Blood, 25
Blood alcohol, 48, 107
  formula, 120
  level, 108-110
Blood-forming organs, 18
Blood level
  data, drug and chemical, 264-271
  lethal, 264
  therapeutic, 264
  toxic, 264
Blood volume, 33
Body cell, 14
Body fat, 25
Body fluids, 22
Body water, 33-34
Bone, 25